Contemporary Diagnosis and Management of

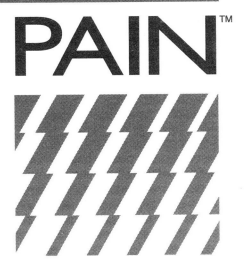

PAIN™

Donlin M. Long, MD
Professor and Chairman of
Neurosurgery
and Founder of the
Pain Treatment Center
Johns Hopkins
Medical Institutions
Baltimore, Maryland

Published by
Handbooks in Health Care Co.,
a division of Associates in Medical Marketing Co., Inc.
Newtown, Pennsylvania, USA

International Standard Book Number: 1-884065-13-9

Library of Congress Catalog Card Number: 96-77897

Contents

This book has been prepared and is presented as a service to the medical community. The information provided reflects the knowledge, experience, and personal opinions of Donlin M. Long, MD, Professor and Chairman of Neurosurgery, Pain Treatment Center, Johns Hopkins Medical Institutions, Baltimore, Maryland.

This book is not intended to replace or to be used as a substitute for the complete prescribing information prepared by each manufacturer for each drug. Because of possible variations in drug indications, in dosage information, in newly described toxicities, in drug/drug interactions, and in other items of importance, reference to such complete prescribing information is definitely recommended before any of the drugs discussed are used or prescribed.

///// Chapter 1

Introduction: Concepts of Pain

Pain as a complication of injury and disease has been a scourge of mankind, as documented in recorded history. The residual evidence of injuries and severe arthritis is found in the remains of Neanderthals. Ancient Egyptian and Greek medical writings discuss pain. Yet almost nothing could be done for the suffering patient until the discovery of opiates. Practical anesthesia is only 150 years old. Local anesthetics have been in common use for barely 100 years, and the broad spectrum of analgesic medications available today is less than 50 years old. Consequently, physicians' ability to manage pain in most diseases has been relatively recent. Therefore, it is not surprising that we do not yet have complete understanding of pain as a complication of disease or injury, or its effects on patients.

Few things a physician does are as important as pain management. We now have the capability to ensure that patients who are injured or ill with pain-producing diseases do not suffer. Pain after surgery can be well controlled. Cancer pain is also treatable for most patients. Despite these capabilities, there is a consensus that pain is not treated as effectively as it might be. The purpose of this book is to provide practicing physicians with a practical way to think about pain problems and to help them provide adequate relief for their suffering patients.

Table 1: Longitudinal Classification of Pain

- **Transient**
    - lasts a short time
    - self-limited

- **Acute**
    - associated with disease
    - postoperative
    - postinjury

- **Persistent**
    - unrelenting with time
    - requires long-term use of analgesics

- **Chronic and Disabling**
    - patients disabled by the pain
    - often accompanied by severe depression and anxiety
    - drug abuse occurs
    - nearly half of all patients have lifelong personality dysfunction

To do this, it is necessary to have a way of thinking about pain that helps govern the philosophical approach to management. One way pain has been described is in terms of duration. Thus, pain is divided by some experts into acute (self-limited) and chronic (will not be improved by waiting). Another classification is based on etiology: cancer pain, postoperative pain, and every other kind of pain lumped into a third large category. Neither of these classifications is satisfactory, but they do have practical significance and can be combined to create a schema to guide the physician in managing pain rationally.

By combining these two classifications we can think about pain longitudinally. In this system, it is generally accepted that pain may be: (1) transient, (2) acute, (3) persistent, or (4) chronic and disabling (Table 1). When thinking about pain in longitudinal terms, it is not necessary to consider etiology, except secondarily. Nor is it necessary to rate pain according to severity, although some clinicians and patients find this approach useful

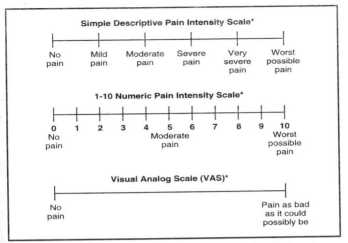

Figure 1: Samples of patient pain intensity scales. * If used as a
graphic rating scale, a 10-cm baseline is recommended.

(Figure 1). We can assume that the pain is severe enough to warrant therapy when the patient seeks relief from a physician. The
real keys to pain management for the physician are to understand what the patient means by pain, to assess how severe and
disabling the pain is, and to decide what reasonable measures
should be used to treat the pain.

Transient pain may be very severe, but its principal characteristic is that it lasts a short time. Typically, transient pain is
self-limited, which makes treatment difficult, perhaps not even
necessary. Understanding the etiology of the pain and treating
any underlying disease are essential. Symptomatic management
for patients suffering from transient recurrent pain is often accomplished with single doses of analgesics and short-term limitation of activities. Treatment with narcotics or other analgesics
is usually acceptable as long as the patient shows no evidence of
drug misuse. More commonly, reassurance that the pain will be
short term is all that is required and no treatment is necessary.[1]

Acute pain complicates injuries and diseases of all kinds.
The most common kinds of acute pain are low back pain and

headache, both of which can last for several days or more. An important subcategory of acute pain is *postoperative pain*. The most important issue in postoperative acute pain is that it will probably disappear by itself. The goal is to keep the patient comfortable during the recuperation period.

Details of acute pain management will follow in the specific chapters. The important thing for clinicians to recognize is that acute pain requires adequate analgesia to make the patient comfortable during the period of recovery. The use of analgesics should be within appropriate medical guidelines, but there is no reason that a patient should suffer unnecessarily during an acute pain episode. Furthermore, there is no reason to fear that the short-term use of narcotics will produce addiction. Adequate analgesia, limitation of activities commensurate with the disease process, and treatment of anxiety that may accompany the disease all are important. Obviously, if there is an underlying disease to be treated, then diagnosis and direct treatment are desirable. The important goals of therapy in the acute pain process are to understand the cause of the pain and to treat that cause while providing adequate analgesia.

Postinjury pain is another subcategory of acute pain. The injury may be obvious, such as a broken bone, or it may be much less obvious, such as in the typical posttraumatic back pain syndrome. The extent and nature of the injury must be evaluated so that reasonable decisions can be made about how long recovery should take and how long analgesia should be provided. There is no way to generalize about how long analgesia should be necessary. It is well known that a broken extremity bone is painful for several weeks, so that 2 to 3 weeks of mild narcotic analgesia is all that is required. On the other hand, a compression fracture of the spine secondary to osteoporosis may produce pain for months, so that long-term narcotics may be required. When soft-tissue injury is all that can be found, then healing within 1 to 2 weeks is usual. Chronic soft-tissue injuries are unlikely.[1]

The most frustrating postinjury issue is disability litigation. It seems probable that the stress of litigation negatively affects the outcome of treatment, but this is rarely an issue in the acute phase of injury. The rules to follow are: complete diagnosis of the injury, appropriate treatment of the injured part, and then analgesia for a reasonable period while healing occurs.[2]

Acute pain complicating other diseases virtually always responds to appropriate treatment of the disease. Here the issues are much more straightforward. Diagnose the disease, treat it appropriately, and provide the patient with enough analgesia to be comfortable while the treatment takes effect. Treatment of the pain should be discontinued as soon as the pain responds to therapy of the disease.

Persistent pain is pain that does not relent with time or even with therapy. Most typical of this kind of pain is low back pain, but virtually any of the pain-producing systemic diseases can also cause persistent pain. The issue for the physician here is quite different. Usually the diagnosis is known, all of the appropriate therapies have been employed, but the patient has not achieved relief. The pain persists. For these patients, the long-term use of analgesics or the use of pain-relieving procedures must be considered. Managing these patients is often difficult and there are many complicating comorbidities that will be discussed under the issue of the chronic pain syndrome. However, the management goal here is straightforward. An appropriate diagnosis is the first step. Then determine whether all of the potentially effective treatments that might cure the underlying problem have been employed. If they have, it is likely that management of the pain will require at least an evaluation by an expert. This usually means referral, first, to an expert in the specific disease, and, second, to an expert in the management of pain. These steps allow for second opinions about the diagnosis and the therapies employed. Then the pain must be treated. The techniques employed vary greatly with the disease. These techniques for specific diseases form the bulk of this book. However, some broad categories of management are available. The use of *long-acting analgesics* is well accepted when the pain is *neoplastic* in origin, but is much less well studied in patients with benign disease. Neurosurgeons use a number of pain-relieving procedures that may be useful, such as cordotomy or spinal stimulation. A *cognitive approach*, which attempts to improve the patient's capacity to deal with a disabling pain syndrome, offers another possibility. A number of important principles must be applied to these patients. *Rigorous diagnosis* is important. While it is necessary to use all appropriate therapies for the underlying disease, there is no reason to repeat them when they have not been beneficial or to try optional therapies that have little chance of success. A *second opinion with an acknowledged expert* is always worthwhile. *Pain-relieving procedures* are valuable for a limited number of specific diseases. Many of these patients can be helped to be more functional by *intensive rehabilitative methods,* especially when the comorbidities that often accompany persistent pain can be treated. Most patients with severe and seriously disabling pain will require evaluation by a pain expert.

The Chronic Pain Syndrome

Some patients are disabled by persistent pain substantially beyond what would be expected from their underlying disease. Some clinicians have defined chronic pain as pain persisting 6 months or more. In addition, they develop serious comorbidities that increase the disability. Typically, patients who exemplify the chronic pain syndrome are disabled by the pain well beyond their physical impairment. Such patients concentrate on the pain, often to the exclusion of everything else, and let pain and pain therapy dominate their lives. Severe depression and chronic anxiety occur. These patients typically undergo numerous fruitless repetitive evaluations and multiple surgeries in the hope of finding a cure. Drug abuse occurs, but true addiction or drug-seeking behavior is relatively uncommon. More typically, these patients simply misuse the drugs, taking narcotics and psychoactive drugs in quantities that substantially impair their functional abilities. Management of chronic pain syndrome is the most difficult of all the various pain problems. In our experience, about one third of these patients have a normal psychiatric history, 15% to 20% have overt psychiatric disease, and the remainder are characterized by lifelong personality dysfunction. Therefore, treatment cannot be for pain alone. It is still important to be certain about the diagnosis and to provide all medical therapies necessary.[3]

However, the greatest benefit to patients with chronic pain syndrome usually comes from identification and treatment of depression and anxiety. Many of these patients are disabled from inactivity and lead very sedentary lives. Their functional capacities can be improved dramatically by antidepressant medications and by vigorous rehabilitative efforts. Drug misuse must be identified and drugs should be prescribed to provide pain relief without seriously affecting mental function. When drug-seeking behavior is identified, it must be corrected. These patients can be protected from additional diagnostic and therapeutic interventions that are not likely to be useful. Some can be restored to function. Unfortunately, a substantial number refuse to accept the realities of their situation and continue searching for the magic cure for pain without being willing to face the importance of the comorbidities in their disability.[4]

The management of chronic pain syndrome requires expert attention, at least in the initial phases. However, it is equally important to have a caring family physician who will regularly reinforce the gains the patient makes from short-term exposure to the pain treatment center.

The *pain treatment center* has evolved over the past 20 years to provide comprehensive management of these comorbidities. To be considered a pain treatment center, the unit should provide: a high-quality, rigorous medical diagnosis; complete psychological/psychiatric evaluation by someone skilled in the treatment of pain; facilities for psychotherapy and drug withdrawal; treatment with antidepressants; use of pain-relieving techniques; and rehabilitation. Without all of these it is unlikely that the comorbidities so common in the chronic pain syndrome can be addressed.

The other etiologic subdivision for chronic pain is pain that occurs with cancer. The medical principles to relieve cancer pain are not dissimilar to those used to relieve pain of other origins. The first goal is always to determine the cause of the pain and treat it. Remember that cancer pain is not always from the neoplastic disease. Rather than making the assumption that the cancer causes the pain, it is important to perform a rigorous diagnosis and then to treat whatever the problem is definitively. Appropriate treatment of the underlying disease usually relieves the pain. However, the use of pain response to judge the value of

Table 2: Common Errors Physicians Make in Managing Patient Pain

- inadequate use of analgesics
- allowing patients to misuse analgesics
- failure to recognize a patient's anxiety and depression, two major contributing factors in pain
- failure to recognize socioeconomic and psychiatric comorbidities
- failure to use available pain therapies

therapy is unacceptable. Pain relief should be immediate and nearly complete. Patients consistently indicate that what they fear most about cancer is unrelieved pain. The goal of management is adequate pain relief without substantial side effects that incapacitate patients or degrade their quality of life. This means beginning treatment with adequate analgesics whenever pain is an issue. Begin with the simplest medications possible. If non-narcotic analgesics suffice, there is no reason to use narcotics. Do not begin with the most potent narcotics; instead, use whatever is adequate to ameliorate the pain and proceed to escalate the dose and change drugs until satisfactory analgesia is obtained. Remember that anxiety and depression can often influence the patient's perception of pain. Both must be appreciated and treated. There is no reason to be concerned about addiction in a patient suffering from pain secondary to advanced cancer. Side effects are the only limits to the use of narcotics for pain control.[5]

Long-Acting Oral Agents

The development of the long-acting oral narcotics has made a dramatic difference in pain control. They can be given in large doses, one, two, or three times per day because they have a long half-life. The absorption rate is small, so the doses required are large. These high doses often frighten inexperienced clinicians in the use of these drugs. However, side effects, not total dose, should be the limiting factor.

The one place destructive procedures are still valuable in pain management is with cancer pain. Intervention should be considered if oral analgesics prove unsatisfactory or if side effects are too serious for the patient to tolerate.

Summary

We may think about pain in terms of etiology, its temporal characteristics, its severity, or a combination of all these factors. The general principles of pain management remain the same. Begin with an accurate diagnosis and treat the underlying disease. Simultaneously provide satisfactory pain control. Once it is clear that pain persists after adequate treatment of the underlying disease, it may be necessary to seek expert advice in pain management. Once that advice is obtained, the ongoing control of the patient's therapy is an important issue and well within the skills of any primary care physician. The most common management errors (Table 2) are: (1) inadequate use of analgesics; (2) allowing patients to misuse these same analgesics; (3) failure to recognize anxiety and depression; (4) failure to recognize socioeconomic and psychiatric comorbidities; and (5) failure to use available pain therapies. All of these are easily correctable. The remainder of this book attempts to help physicians eliminate these management errors from medical practice.

References

1. Cailliet R: *Soft Tissue Pain and Disability*. Philadelphia, FA Davis Co, 1977.

2. Sternbach RA, ed. *The Psychology of Pain.* 2nd ed. New York, Raven Press, 1986.

3. France RD, Krishnan KRR: Pain in psychiatric disorders. In: France RD, Krishnan KRR, eds. *Chronic Pain.* Washington, American Psychiatric Press, 1988, pp 116-141.

4. Pilowsky I, Chapman CR, Bonica JJ: Pain, depression and illness behavior in a pain clinic population. *Pain* 1977;4:183-192.

5. Portenoy RK: Cancer pain: epidemiology and syndromes. *Cancer* 1989;63(S):2298-2307.

Chapter 2

Anatomy and Physiology of Pain

The sensation of pain depends on the activation of a discreet group of receptors and their fibers, on ascending tracts, on cells and neurons in the brain stem, on the thalamus, and on the cerebral cortex (Figure 1). Scientific knowledge of the processing of pain information has increased enormously in the past 30 years. We now know, for example, that a variety of arousal, somatic, autonomic, and affective reactions occur with pain.

Pain results when noxious stimuli activate *nociceptors*, which are pain receptors in the skin. The pain sensation is conducted from the receptor through fine fibers called A delta and C in peripheral nerves. The cell bodies for these receptors are located in spinal *dorsal root ganglia* and connect with the *dorsal horn* of the spinal cord. Conduction of pain depends on axons ascending in the *anterolateral quadrant* on the side of the body opposite to the nociceptor. Higher processing of pain involves the *thalamus* and the *cerebral cortex*. There are many interactions in the brain stem. The pain system is widely connected to the limbic system, which may account for the affective component of pain. Understanding the anatomy and neuropharmacology of the pain system has led to the development of stimulation techniques for pain control, new diagnostic tests, and new analgesic drugs.[1]

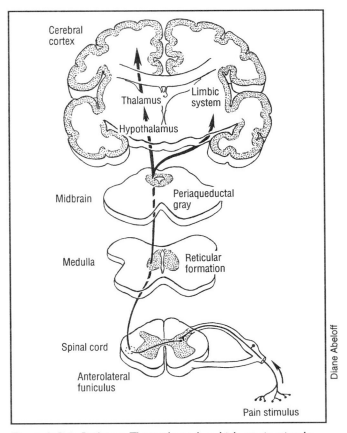

Figure 1: Pain Pathway. The pathway by which a pain stimulus enters consciousness begins in the periphery with the receptor whose cell body is located in the dorsal horn. Synapses are made in the ipsilateral dorsal horn. Pain fibers cross to the opposite side of the spinal cord to ascend in the anterolateral funiculus. Many connections in the reticular system and the brain stem relate to the reflex changes associated with pain. Multiple connections with the limbic system and hypothalamus account for the emotional changes of pain. Synapses occur in the thalamus and are projected to the cortex and the consciousness.

15

Nociceptors

Specific areas of sensation in the nervous system were discovered about 100 years ago. These include areas specific for touch, warmth, cold, and pain. Also, specific nerve terminals were found to serve each sensation. There are two main classes of nociceptors: those that respond to mechanical stimulation (A delta) and those that respond to many sensations (C). Cutaneous pain sensation has two specific qualities: a pin-prick sensation and another sensation usually described as burning. The sharp, pricking pain is the result of excitation of A delta nociceptors; the burning pain is the result of excitation of C nociceptors. Painful stimuli produce a first and second pain. The pricking pain is felt first; the burning pain lasts longer and is not localized, but diffuse.

Another important concept in the pain process is hyperalgesia. Hyperalgesia is spontaneous pain that often follows damage to the skin. There is a reduced pain threshold around the area of injury, called *primary hyperalgesia*. A surrounding area of undamaged skin may develop *secondary hyperalgesia*. The secondary effect is important because it results in widespread pain, swelling, and stiffness that often far exceeds the original pain at the area of injury. Excitatory chemicals such as somatostatin and substance P, as well as sensitizing chemicals such as bradykinin and prostaglandin, occur in the peripheral receptors and other tissues. Some researchers have postulated that the release of these chemicals from damaged cells is important in the process that activates nociceptors. This theory is still unproven. In addition to skin, nociceptors are found in muscle and joints. They also occur in the viscera, but the distribution and actions of visceral nociceptors have not been extensively studied.

In addition to the principal nociceptors, the A delta and C, new receptors called *sleeping* or *silent* have recently been described. These nociceptors do not react to mechanical stimuli. They become active only when tissue is injured and thereby add to the known nociceptive input to the nervous system. They then acquire mechanical sensitivity and, in turn, add to hyperalgesia. The primary hyperalgesia, which develops locally in the area of injury, is secondary to sensitization of all the nociceptors. The secondary hyperalgesia that spreads is secondary to central hyperexcitability. Allodynia also develops. This is defined as perception of pain in response to a stimulus that is normally not pain producing. Allodynia is commonly misunderstood as a psychiatric symptom.[2]

Sensitization

No single substance is known to produce sensitization; instead, a mixture of substances contributes to this process. A major part of sensitization is the awakening of the *sleeping* nociceptors. The clinical consequences include exaggerated responses to stimuli applied in the periphery and an increase in the area from which such responses can be produced. The sensitization and convergence of input explain referred pain. The classic example occurs with myocardial ischemia, which produces substernal pressure, chest and shoulder radiation, and, occasionally, arm and neck radiation. The skin on the chests of these patients becomes hyperalgesic.[2]

Nociceptive Input to the Dorsal Horn

Once the peripheral pain receptors (nociceptors) are activated, the pain sensation travels along the thinly myelinated A delta fibers or the unmyelinated C fibers to the dorsal root ganglion, where the cell bodies of these neurons are located. Sensation is then transmitted through the dorsal roots to the dorsal horn. One of the great anatomical discoveries is attributed to Bell and Magendie, who described the sensory function of the dorsal roots and the motor function of the ventral roots. As the sensory fibers in the dorsal roots approach the spinal cord, the fine pain-carrying fibers are found laterally and the larger nonpain fibers aggregate medially. The pain fibers enter the spinal cord superficial to the dorsal horn and run up and down in a tract (Lissauer's) that provides connections over many segments. In addition to these posterior fibers, we now know that ventral roots contain many afferent fibers. The peripheral receptive fields associated with these fibers are often nociceptive. This finding has been used to explain the observation that dorsal rhizotomy is not an effective way to control pain.

The primary afferent fibers enter the substantia gelatinosa on its dorsal aspect. These pain-carrying fibers end in several layers of the dorsal horn. Substance P and a number of other peptides are found in these areas. As yet, these chemicals cannot be identified with specific classes of receptors. The detailed anatomy of the innumerable interactions that occur in the dorsal horn has been the subject of much research and is now understood in greater detail. In humans, most of the fibers in the pain system cross in the anterior commissure of the spinal cord anterior to the central canal and ascend as the lateral spinothalamic tract on the opposite side of the spinal cord.

Ascending Nociceptive Tracts

The lateral spinothalamic tract ascending in the anterolateral quadrant is the most important spinal cord pain tract in humans. The tract reaches from the insertion of the dentate ligament to the ventral roots. There is a somatotopic relationship with sacral fibers located superficially and closest to the dentate ligament. The cervical fibers are aggregated medially. In addition to this specific tract, spinoreticular and spinomesencephalic systems are also nociceptive. Little is known about these systems in humans. The spinothalamic system gives off collaterals in the brain stem to the reticular formation and the periaqueductal gray. The spinothalamic system ascends through the brain stem just above the inferior olivary nucleus and then is adjacent to the lateral lemniscus. This tract terminates in the ventral posterior lateral nucleus of the thalamus (VPL). There is a somatotopic relationship of the terminations in this nucleus, and terminations in the reticular portion of the thalamus as well. Thalamic connections in the limbic system probably explain motivational affective aspects of pain. A cortical representation for pain receives direct transmissions from these thalamic areas.

Nociceptive Transmission to Cerebral Cortex

For many years it was generally accepted that cortical stimulation did not cause pain. However, research has confirmed that stimulation of the cerebral cortex in humans does sometimes produce pain and that destructive lesions of the postcentral gyrus may reduce pain. Pain is occasionally a part of an epileptic aura and the so-called thalamic pain syndrome can be caused by lesions of the cortex that have not caused any direct injury to the thalamus. The VPL nucleus, which is the termination of the spinothalamic tract, projects both to primary and secondary sensory regions of the cortex. While cortical representation in humans is generally well accepted now, the exact anatomy and physiology of the cortical interactions are not well understood.

Descending Inhibitory Systems

A descending system seems to involve medial and reticular thalamus, the periaqueductal gray, a number of brain stem nuclear centers, and a fiber tract that descends in the lateral dorsal spinal cord to interact with nociceptive dorsal horn cells. The presence of this descending system and its inhibitory influences are well accepted in some animal species. Their presence in humans is not certain.

The Gate Control Theory

The concept of sensory interaction was introduced by Melzack and Wall[3] and is generally termed *the gate control theory*. Gate control implies the ability of one part of the nonpain sensory system to inhibit or intensify transmission in the pain pathways. The discovery of these control mechanisms led to the development of spinal cord stimulators and other forms of nervous system stimulation for pain control.

Opioid Receptors and the Internal Opiate System

Pert and Snyder[4] first described the receptors on nerve cells that bind opiates, thereby explaining the analgesic effects of narcotics. Several kinds of receptors exist and each has specific properties. The location of these cells has been extensively studied.

The many advances in the pain process have expanded our understanding of pain and the system that conducts it in humans. Future research will provide us with more information about other substances, such as substance P, somatostatin, and bradykinin, to name a few, that are involved in pain transmission. The specific relationship of these substances to specific pain syndromes is unclear. Antagonists that might supplant narcotics are theoretically possible, but none has been developed yet that is effective.

New Approaches to Pain Management

Increased understanding of the anatomy of pain has led to a series of new and promising approaches. Among these is excitatory amino-acid receptor antagonists, several of which are under study. Another approach is based on some evidence that premedication with opioids will reduce sensitization, which can be particularly useful in postsurgical patients. Opioid agonists, which would activate opioid receptors, are also targets for the development of analgesic compounds. None is available at present, but this new class of drugs is being vigorously explored. Another class of compounds, called delta peptides, is under investigation. Research has shown that occupation of the delta receptors potentiates the action of opioids. Therefore, these drugs may improve the pain relief obtained from opioids.[2]

Among the novel approaches to pain control, studies are determining if it may be possible to implant analgesic-releasing cells in the region of the spinal cord. These cells create analgesic compounds and act as pumps to deliver them into the spinal canal. Some researchers have proposed that this method can prevent the synthesis of receptor proteins in the pain pathways, compared to traditional methods of trying to create blockades in those pathways.

References

1. Willis WD: The pain system—the neural basis of nociceptive transmission in the mammalian nervous system. In: Gildenberg PL, ed. *Pain and Headache*. Basel (Switzerland), Karger, 1985, vol 8.

2. Therapeutic developments in pain control. Study guide. American Pain Society Audioprogram. MPE Communications Inc, Fair Lawn, NJ, December, 1995.

3. Melzack R, Wall PD: Pain mechanisms: a new theory. *Science* 1965;150:971-979.

4. Pert CB, Snyder SH: Opiate receptor: demonstration in nervous tissue. *Science* 1973;179:1011-1014.

Chapter 3

Management of Postinjury and Postoperative Pain

P ain is an unavoidable consequence of serious injuries and of most surgery. The initial pain of tissue injury is soon complicated by an inflammatory process and expanded by transient changes in the sensitivity of central neurons. Postinjury pain is usually severe for 48 hours, significant for about 5 days, and then gradually disappears 2 to 3 weeks after injury. In most longitudinal studies, patients need continuous analgesia for 2 to 5 days. After that, episodic analgesia taken by the patient as needed is adequate.

Consequences of Postoperative Pain

Unrelieved postoperative pain has several negative consequences beyond the patient's suffering. The stress response is immediate, corticotropin (ACTH) is increased, and there is a substantial endorphin release. The stresses on the heart can be significant, but can be avoided by adequate analgesia. In addition, patients in pain often become immobile. Muscle wasting is rapid, joints stiffen, and the incidence of thromboembolism increases. Patients with abdominal and thoracic incisions may not breathe well and respiratory complications may therefore ensue. For all these reasons, adequate postoperative analgesia is of major importance.[1]

Table 1: Opioids and Their Characteristics

Sustained-release morphine sulfate (SRMS)

- SRMS contains morphine in a matrix of aliphatic alcohol, cellulose, and lactose (MS Contin®, Oramorph SR™).
- Typical dosing is q 12 h; however, more frequent (q 8 h) dosing may be needed in patients with AIDS because of higher metabolic rate and poor absorption.

Methadone

- This agent (Dolophine®) is highly lipid soluble and long acting. Its analgesic half-life is about 6 h, its oral bioavailability is close to 90%.
- It may be an effective alternative for persons who are morphine-intolerant.
- Accumulation can occur with acute (q 4 h) dosing, with subsequent side effects (sedation, respiratory depression).
- Concomitant use of rifampin or phenytoin can increase methadone metabolism and shorten its analgesic effect.[1]

Analgesics for Acute Postoperative and Postinjury Pain

The most important issue in postoperative pain management is the appropriate use of analgesics, both nonnarcotic and opioid agents (Table 1). The standards are oral and parenteral narcotics. (A comparison of equivalent dosages and durations of action is provided in Tables 2, 3, 4, and 5 in Chapter 4.) The key clinical principles are to use enough of whatever agent is chosen and to give the drug often enough to achieve prolonged analgesia. Typically, patients require parenteral narcotics for 48 hours after most major surgery and then can be switched to oral drugs. The dose of narcotic can be slowly reduced over several days; most patients need only episodic oral narcotics 5 to 7 days after surgery.

The major problems with this standard regimen are in timing the narcotic administration and in not recognizing when to administer the drugs. The p.r.n. use of narcotics in the average hospital is associated with several problems. The patient waits until the pain becomes reasonably severe before asking the nurse for pain medication. There is then a delay of 20 to 40 minutes before the drug arrives, and a further delay of about 20 minutes after administration before reasonable analgesia occurs. Because maximal analgesia with most narcotics lasts about 90 minutes before a decline in efficacy begins, such a regimen produces peaks of adequate analgesia and valleys of inadequate analgesia. Reputable studies suggest that the average patient receives pain relief only about half the time in such a regimen. These problems can be overcome by administering the drugs more frequently and by educating all health-care personnel to understand the importance of prompt analgesic administration when needed.[2]

A way to improve the duration of analgesia is to give the drug at regular intervals rather than on a p.r.n. basis. This strategy provides adequate blood levels that persist. It is important to be certain that accumulation of the narcotic does not occur. Therefore, all involved need to be aware of the common side effects of narcotic overdose: confusion followed by somnolence, reduced respiratory rate, reduced blood pressure, and reduced heart rate.

Patient-Controlled Analgesia

The newest regimen that attempts to eliminate the vagaries of the time-honored system of nurse/patient interaction is patient-controlled analgesia.[3] The narcotics are placed in intravenous solution and a small computer or other dispensing device monitors a prescribed amount of the drug. The patient self-administers the analgesic whenever pain occurs. Overdose is prevented by governing the amount of drug that can be given and, theoretically, this almost continuous infusion maintains an adequate blood level, reduces patients' dependence on other personnel, and gives them a sense of control over the pain. Patients are generally satisfied with this approach. However, the outcome of patient-controlled analgesia as measured by pain control is not as good as we would like. For example, when patients go to sleep, medication is not given, the pain rears up, and they often awake in severe pain. Elderly and confused patients sometimes cannot use the devices effectively. Side effects are substantially more common than with analgesics administered by a nurse. The principal risk is respiratory depression. In general, patient-controlled analgesia should not be used with patients undergoing craniotomy or cervical operations above the C5 level. Elderly and debilitated patients do not tolerate it well.[3,4]

There are many devices on the market. If this technique is to be used, the establishment of a postoperative pain service should be considered. The devices and the patients must be monitored regularly to assure that pain control is satisfactory and that side effects are minimized.

Transdermal analgesia is another available technique. Fentanyl patches (Duragesic®) are very effective for many patients and eliminate the need for repeated dosing.[5]

Spinal Opiates for Postoperative Pain

The epidural or intrathecal administration of opiates is another technique that can be very useful.[6] Regional epidural analgesia can provide excellent anesthesia for thoracotomy incision or abdominal incision. The technique has been less useful for laminectomy. To use the technique, a spinal catheter is inserted near the segments where analgesia is to be obtained. If analgesia is required for an extremity incision, it should be placed in the general area where the roots to be anesthetized exit the spinal canal. Water-soluble morphine is the most common drug used. Remember that a pyrogen-free drug is required for intrathecal administration. The lipid-soluble drugs, fentanyl and sufentanil, are also used.

The catheters are placed when surgery is complete and the drugs are administered regularly to provide analgesia. When epidural anesthesia is used, the same catheter is simply left in place. This is the most common technique. The issues of administration are adequate analgesia and adverse side effects. The most common reason for failure is movement of the catheter, preventing the drug from reaching the appropriate segments. Adverse effects include respiratory depression, nausea, pleuritis, and urinary retention, all of which are serious. When patients are treated with spinal opiates all personnel involved in their care must understand the management of an indwelling catheter and must follow a monitoring program for side effects, particularly respiratory depression.[1,2]

Local Anesthetic Techniques for Pain Control

Peripheral nerve blocks are among the oldest techniques to control postoperative pain. Two common techniques are now in use. Intercostal blocks following thoracotomy provide long-lasting relief of thoracotomy pain. Blockade of the nerve near a chest tube is also an important technique. Continuous plexus block for the relief of pain secondary to an extremity incision is another excellent technique. The adverse side effects are sensitivity to the agent used and the motor sensory deficit brought on by the plexus blockade. Local anesthetic toxicity is an issue. These patients must be monitored carefully for hypotension, urinary retention, toxicity, and the effects of the motor sensory block.

Intrapleural Analgesia

Another technique that satisfactorily relieves post-thoracotomy pain is the use of an indwelling catheter placed within the pleura in the region of the surgery. The same drugs are employed that might be used for epidural analgesia. Dose and frequency of administration will depend on the drug chosen and the analgesia to be obtained. There is an increased risk of pneumothorax; also, local anesthetic toxicity is a problem.

Transcutaneous Electrical Nerve Stimulation

Evidence suggests that transcutaneous electrical nerve stimulation applied in the area surrounding the incision will provide adequate postoperative analgesia without any of the side effects of narcotics. The low cost, lack of side effects, and the patient's ability to control the stimulation all make this an attractive technique to pursue. Yet, despite reports in the literature that support its use, this technique has never achieved much popularity. This is probably because there are few centers where it can be efficiently employed. Like patient-controlled analgesia of any other kind, its effective use requires the development of a postoperative pain service to provide for maintenance of the equipment, patient education, and monitoring of effect.[7]

Summary

Adequate techniques are available for the effective control of postoperative pain. The physician's goal is to eliminate all pain as far as possible without any dangerous or unpleasant side effects. Given the techniques available, there is little reason why any patient should suffer serious postoperative or postinjury pain. The short-term use of narcotics does not carry a risk of addiction. In fact, the fear of addiction, which is so common among health-care personnel, is unfounded. Give the patient adequate analgesia that minimizes side effects. However, remember that postoperative pain usually ceases within 2 to 3 weeks and that the long-standing use of narcotics after surgery is unwarranted for most patients. Persisting pain usually indicates a complication or reflects psychological factors that need attention. The patient who requires prolonged use of narcotics after surgery needs re-evaluation rather than simple continuation of the drugs.

References

1. Bromage PR, Camporesi E, Chestnut D: Epidural narcotics for postoperative analgesia. *Anesth Analg* 1980;59:473.

2. Cousins MJ, Bridenbaugh PO: Spinal opioids and pain relief in acute care. In: Cousins MJ, Philips GD, eds. *Acute Pain Management.* New York, Churchill Livingstone, 1986, pp 151-185.

3. Harmer M, Rosen M, Vickers MD, eds. *Patient-Controlled Analgesia.* Oxford, Blackwell Scientific Publications, 1985.

4. Mather LE, Owen H: The scientific basis of patient-controlled analgesia. *Anesth Intens Care* 1988;16:427-447.

5. Varvel JR, Shafer SL, Hwang SS, et al: Absorption characteristics of transdermally administered fentanyl. *Anesthesiology* 1989;70:928-934.

6. Covino BA, Lambert DH: Epidural and spinal anesthesia. In: Barash PG, Cullen BF, Stoelting RK, eds. *Clinical Anesthesia.* Philadelphia, JB Lippincott, 1989, pp 755-786.

7. Solomon RA, Viernstein MC, Long DM: Reduction of postoperative pain and narcotic use by transcutaneous electrical nerve stimulation. *Surgery* 1980;87:142.

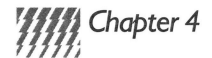 *Chapter 4*

Management of Cancer Pain

Pain complicating cancer may be a direct effect of the tumor or secondary to tumor treatment or to an unrelated disease. The clinician's first step is to make an accurate diagnosis. Before automatically resorting to narcotics, clinicians must identify the cause so they can prescribe appropriate therapy in addition to pain relief.[1]

Identifying the cause has major practical importance. If pain is a direct effect of the tumor, then appropriate therapy is tumor treatment and pain relief. Pain relief alone is used only when no additional cancer therapy is required or possible or when no concurrent disease is found.

The pathophysiology of each cancer pain syndrome has important implications for therapy. The most common cause of pain is when a tumor activates the normal nociceptive system. Tumor invasion or pressure from an expanding tumor, associated infection or inflammation, and bony collapse are all typical tumor effects that cause pain. Visceral pain is more commonly from bowel or ureteral obstruction. Direct treatment of the cancer and relief of secondary effects, such as bowel obstruction, are primary. Pain relief should be simultaneous. Some have advocated measuring the value of therapy by the effect on pain; it is far better to give the patient adequate analgesics and then gradually reduce medications as the effect of therapy becomes apparent.

27

Neuropathic pain results from injury to the nervous system. Neuropathic syndromes are unusual, but they are important to recognize because their treatment is quite different from disease states that trigger pain in a normal nervous system. Three forms of neuropathic pain are common. The most typical are neuropathies following neurotoxic chemotherapy. These patients develop paresthesias, dysesthesias, and pain associated with sensory loss in the extremities. The neuropathy usually has a stocking-glove distribution and may be associated with motor loss as well. The stocking-glove sensory loss and the known chemotherapy are adequate to make the diagnosis, which can be substantiated by electromyography. The usual treatment is to reduce the level of chemotherapy.

Neuropathy and the other neuropathic pains may respond to specific drugs not commonly considered to be analgesics. Drugs that can be useful for these patients include carbamazepine (Tegretol®) administered in escalating doses from 200 mg/day to 800 mg/day; amitriptyline (Elavil®) 25 mg/day to 100 mg/day; and clonazepam (Klonopin®) 1.5 mg/day. The common side effects of carbamazepine are confusion, fatigue, and somnolence. Amitriptyline may have those same effects as well as dry mouth and constipation. Confusion and somnolence are the most common side effects of clonazepam, which can also have an alerting effect occasionally. Narcotics are not useful for most neuropathic pain.

Deafferentation pain results when a lesion occurs in the pain pathway in the central nervous system, usually in the thalamus, or when tumor invasion and destruction occur in the primary afferent fibers. Typical examples would be tumor invasion of lumbosacral or brachial plexus. The pain is usually continuous, may be aggravated by emotion, and is perceived in the distribution of the involved fibers or in a body part represented by the area of thalamus destroyed. The pain tends to be widespread. Thalamic pain, for example, usually involves an entire side of the body. Deafferentation pain is usually associated with a sensory disturbance; paralysis may or may not be present. This pain is particularly disturbing to patients because there is often a distortion of perception so that nonpainful stimuli, such as a light touch or change in temperature, may trigger intense pain. These pains respond to the same classes of medications as does neuropathic pain.

Sympathetically maintained pain, more commonly called *reflex sympathetic dystrophy* or *RSD*, is a special category of pain just beginning to be understood. The pain is neuropathic in origin, but there is an interaction with the sympathetic nervous system. Hyperesthesia or sensitivity to light touch are common manifestations. The extremity is usually cold, may be swollen, and does not sweat. Less commonly, the extremity may be warm and sweat excessively. The diagnosis is made when the pain is eliminated by sympathetic blockade. Surgical sympathectomy has been the traditional treatment and it is very effective. Endoscopic and percutaneous sympathectomies have been described and chemical sympathectomy is possible. Whenever this diagnosis is suspected, the sympathetic blockade should be diagnostic.

A similar pain syndrome, a particular form of deafferentation pain, is not related to the sympathetic nervous system. Even though the two may seem to be identical clinically, the sympathetically independent pain does not respond to sympathetic blockade. It may respond to the classes of medications used for other neuropathic pain.[2]

Factors Other Than Pain That Influence Treatment

Patients with cancer routinely become anxious and depressed. It is not uncommon for a patient who has failed to achieve pain relief with substantial doses of narcotics to nonetheless improve with adequate treatment of depression. Anxiety also may require treatment. Some patients who have responded well to treatment of the primary tumor may develop such a cancer neurosis that the pain persists because of psychological factors. Whenever a patient fails to respond to appropriate analgesic therapy, it is worthwhile reassessing the possibility of psychological factors.

Because of its substantial duration, cancer pain control depends on support systems available to the patient. First, there must be an understanding physician who appreciates the pain and understands the appropriate use of analgesics. Next, financial considerations are important. Many of the long-acting narcotics are expensive. Some of the techniques require that the patient have family members or others in the social system to help with medications or device control. Side effects of the medication may be amplified by tumor therapy. For example, treatment of primary tumors commonly causes asthenia and constipation, both of which are side effects of narcotic medications. Nausea commonly occurs with chemotherapy and may interfere with the use of oral narcotics.[2]

The Goal of Cancer Pain Therapy

The first goal of cancer therapy is pain relief (Figure 1). If the patient has other distressing symptoms or side effects from the medication, these must be treated as well. Nausea is the most common. The overall goal is to keep the patient functioning independently and pain free.[3]

Analgesics in Cancer

The cancer pain therapist must know the temporal pattern and severity of the patient's pain. If the pain is continuous, then a system of continuous analgesia with stable blood levels is required. If the patient has acute episodes superimposed upon a continuous pain pattern, then as-needed doses of analgesics may be required for breakthrough pain. When the pain is acute but intermittent, then as-needed medications are preferred.

The severity of the pain determines the type of treatment. When the pain is mild, begin with nonnarcotic analgesics. These include aspirin, acetaminophen (Tylenol®), and the broad spectrum of nonsteroidal anti-inflammatory drugs (NSAIDs) (Table 1). These drugs may be used in combination with an occasional opioid. Because of their peripheral anti-inflammatory effects, they are particularly useful for pain secondary to bone invasion.

Moderate pain requires opioids. Begin with codeine, oxycodone (Percodan®, Roxicodone™, Tylox®), and propoxyphene (Darvocet®, Darvon®). These drugs are often used with a nonnarcotic analgesic. They have few side effects. When one of these drugs proves ineffective, a clinician can simply switch to another rather than moving to those opioids that are employed for severe cancer pain. The typical doses are found in Tables 2 and 3.

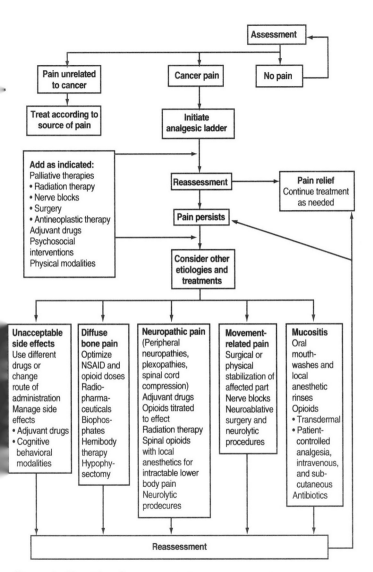

Figure 1: Algorithm for cancer pain management.

31

Table 1: Dosing Data for Acetaminophen and NSAIDs

Drug	Usual dose for adults ≥ 50 kg body weight
Acetaminophen and over-the-counter NSAIDs	
Acetaminophen[2] (Excedrin®, Percogesic®, Tylenol®)	650 mg q 4 h 975 mg q 6 h
Aspirin[3]	650 mg q 4 h 975 mg q 6 h
Ibuprofen (Advil®, Bayer®, Motrin®)	400-600 mg q 6 h
Prescription NSAIDs	
Carprofen (Rimadyl®)	100 mg t.i.d.
Choline magnesium trisalicylate[4] (Trilisate®)	1,000-1,500 mg t.i.d.
Choline salicylate (Arthropan®)[4]	870 mg q 3-4 h
Diflunisal (Dolobid®)[5]	500 mg q 12 h
Etodolac (Lodine®)	200-400 mg q 6-8 h

[1]Acetaminophen and NSAID dosages for adults weighing less than 50 kg should be adjusted for weight.
[2]Acetaminophen lacks the peripheral anti-inflammatory and antiplatelet activities of the other NSAIDs.
[3]The standard against which other NSAIDs are compared. May inhibit platelet aggregation for a week and may cause bleeding.
[4]May have minimal antiplatelet activity.
[5]Administration with antacids may decrease absorption.

**Usual dose for adults
<50 kg body weight[1]**

10-15 mg/kg q 4 h
15-20 mg/kg q 4 h (rectal)

10-15 mg/kg q 4 h
15-20 mg/kg q 4 h (rectal)

10 mg/kg q 6-8 h

25 mg/kg t.i.d.

Note: Only the above NSAIDs have FDA approval for use as simple analgesics, but clinical experience has been gained with other drugs as well.

Codes: q=every   t.i.d.=three times daily

(continued on next page)

Table 1: Dosing Data for Acetaminophen and NSAIDs *(continued)*

Drug	Usual dose for adults ≥ 50 kg body weight
Fenoprofen calcium (Nalfon®)	300-600 mg q 6 h
Ketoprofen (Orudis®)	25-60 mg q 6-8 h
Ketorolac tromethamine[6] (Toradol®)	10 mg q 4-6 h to a maximum of 40 mg/day
Magnesium salicylate (Doan's®, Magan®, Mobidin®, others)	650 mg q 4 h
Meclofenamate sodium (Meclomen®)[7]	50-100 mg q 6 h
Mefenamic acid (Ponstel®)	250 mg q 6 h
Naproxen (Naprosyn®)	250-275 mg q 6-8 h
Naproxen sodium (Aleve®, Anaprox®)	275 mg q 6-8 h
Sodium salicylate (generic)	325-650 mg q 3-4 h
Parenteral NSAIDs	
Ketorolac tromethamine[6,8] (Toradol®)	60 mg initially, then 30 mg q 6 h Intramuscular dose not to exceed 5 days

When cancer pain becomes severe, the drugs typically used are morphine (MS Contin®, MSIR®, Oramorph SR™, Roxanol™), methadone (Dolophine®), levorphanol (Levo-Dromoran®), hydromorphone (Dilaudid®), oxycodone (Roxicodone™), and transdermal fentanyl (Duragesic®). Meperidine (Demerol®) has a toxic metabolite and is not used much in cancer treatment. It is an excellent postoperative analgesic, but the presence of the toxic metabolite makes its long-term use less desirable.

Oral and/or transdermal analgesics should be used as long as possible. For this reason, methadone, oxycodone, hydro-

**Usual dose for adults
<50 kg body weight**[1]

5 mg/kg q 8 h

[6]For short-term use only.
[7]Coombs-positive autoimmune hemolytic anemia has been associated with prolonged use.
[8]Has the same GI toxicities as oral NSAIDs.

morphone, transdermal fentanyl (Duragesic®), and the newly developed long-acting forms of morphine (MS Contin® and Oramorph SR™) are desirable. The typical doses and durations of action are found in Tables 2, 3, and 6.

Specific Management of Analgesics in Cancer

Begin with a nonnarcotic analgesic at reasonable doses and continue for as long as pain control is satisfactory. If the pain escapes, try changing to another nonnarcotic analgesic. If this is ineffective, add a mild opioid such as codeine or oxycodone.

Table 2: Dose Equivalents for Opioid Analgesics in Opioid-naive Adults ≥ 50 kg[1]

Drug	Approximate equianalgesic dose	
	Oral	Parenteral
opioid agonist[2]		
Morphine[3,4] (MSIR®, Roxanol™)	30 mg q 3-4 h (repeat around-the-clock dosing)	10 mg q 3-4 h
	60 mg q 3-4 h (single dose or intermittent dosing)	
Morphine, controlled-release[3,4] (MS Contin®, Oramorph SR™)	90-120 mg q 12 h	N/A
Hydromorphone[3,4] (Dilaudid®)	7.5 mg q 3-4 h	1.5 mg q 3-4 h
Levorphanol (Levo-Dromoran®)	4 mg q 6-8 h	2 mg q 6-8 h
Meperidine[4,5] (Demerol®)	300 mg q 2-3 h	100 mg q 3 h
Methadone (Dolophine®)	20 mg q 6-8 h	10 mg q 6-8 h
Oxymorphone[3,4] (Numorphan®)	N/A	1 mg q 3-4 h

[1]Caution: Recommended doses do not apply for adult patients with body weight less than 50 kg. For recommended starting doses for adults <50 kg body weight, see Table 3.

[2]Caution: Recommended doses do not apply to patients with renal or hepatic insufficiency or other conditions affecting drug metabolism and kinetics.

[3]Caution: For morphine, hydromorphone, and oxymorphone, rectal administration is an alternate route for patients unable to take oral medications. Equianalgesic doses may differ from oral and parenteral doses because of pharmacokinetic differences.

[4]Transdermal fentanyl (Duragesic®) is an alternative. See Table 6. See package insert for dosing calculations. Doses above 25 μg/h should not be used in opioid-naive patients.

| **Usual starting dose for moderate to severe pain** | |
Oral	Parenteral
30 mg q 3-4 h	10 mg q 3-4 h
90-120 mg q 12 h	N/A
6 mg q 3-4 h	1.5 mg q 3-4 h
4 mg q 6-8 h	2 mg q 6-8 h
N/R	100 mg q 3 h
20 mg q 6-8 h	10 mg q 6-8 h
N/A	1 mg q 3-4 h

[5]Not recommended. Doses listed are for brief therapy. Switch to another opioid for long-term therapy.
[6]Caution: Doses of aspirin and acetaminophen in combination opioid/NSAID preparations must also be adjusted to the patient's body weight.
[7]Caution: Codeine doses above 65 mg often are not appropriate because of diminishing incremental analgesia and continually increasing nausea, constipation, and other side effects.

N/A = not available.
N/R = not recommended.

(continued on next page)

Table 2: Dose Equivalents for Opioid Analgesics in Opioid-naive Adults ≥ 50 kg[1]

(continued)

Drug	Approximate equianalgesic dose	
	Oral	**Parenteral**
Combination opioid/ NSAID preparations[6]		
Codeine (with aspirin or acetaminophen)[7] (Capital® with Codeine, Phenaphen®, Tylenol® with Codeine)	180-200 mg q 3-4 h	130 mg q 3-4 h
Hydrocodone (Lorcet®, Lortab®, Vicodin®)	30 mg q 3-4 h	N/A
Oxycodone (Percocet®, Percodan®, Roxicodone™, Tylox®)	30 mg q 3-4 h	N/A

These are particularly useful because they are combined with nonnarcotic analgesics in a single tablet. Escalate the dose until side effects occur or until pain relief proves inadequate. Then move to the longer-acting oral or transdermal narcotics. Methadone is an excellent choice because it needs to be administered only 2 or 3 times per day and it is inexpensive compared to most other choices. Other techniques should be considered only when the oral or transdermal routes of administration have failed.

Most oral opioids require dosing every 3 to 4 hours round the clock to achieve adequate relief of moderate or severe pain. Less serious pain can usually be managed on an as-needed basis. However, when pain is substantial, the round-the-clock schedule is desirable. Methadone usually can be given every 6 to 8 hours and controlled-release morphine needs to be given only every 8 to 12 hours. If the dosing schedule used is strictly p.r.n., the patient will have substantial periods when pain control is not satisfactory. Round-the-

Usual starting dose for moderate to severe pain	
Oral	**Parenteral**
60 mg q 3-4 h	60 mg q 2 h (IM/SC)
10 mg q 3-4 h	N/A
10 mg q 3-4 h	N/A

clock dosing on a schedule is preferable. However, breakthrough pain can occur and the patient needs to be offered the opportunity for additional medication on an as-needed basis for it. The right dose of the opioid is not fixed; it is whatever is required to provide analgesia without side effects.

Clinicians must also understand the formulas when converting from oral to parenteral opioids (Tables 4 and 5); or from oral and IM opioids to transdermal opioid (Table 6).

Some physicians and nurses persist in being concerned about the addiction potential of narcotics in these patients. This fear is unwarranted. Addiction is a psychological and behavioral disorder characterized by drug seeking. True addiction virtually never occurs during opioid treatment for cancer pain unless the patient has a history of addiction before the need for cancer pain therapy. The habituation that does occur is not disabling and should not interfere with the appropriate use of narcotics for adequate pain control.

Table 3: Dose Equivalents for Opioid Analgesics in Opioid-naive Adults <50 kg

Drug	Approximate equianalgesic dose	
	Oral	Parenteral
opioid agonist[1]		
Morphine[2,3] (MSIR®, Roxanol™)	30 mg q 3-4 h (repeat around-the-clock dosing)	10 mg q 3-4 h
	60 mg q 3-4 h (single dose or intermittent dosing)	
Morphine, controlled-release[2,3] (MS Contin®, Oramorph SR™)	90-120 mg q 12 h	N/A
Hydromorphone[2,3] (Dilaudid®)	7.5 mg q 3-4 h	1.5 mg q 3-4 h
Levorphanol (Levo-Dromoran®)	4 mg q 6-8 h	2 mg q 6-8 h
Meperidine[3,4] (Demerol®)	300 mg q 2-3 h	100 mg q 3
Methadone[3] (Dolophine®, others)	20 mg q 6-8 h	10 mg q 6-8 h
Combination opioid/NSAID preparations[5]		
Codeine[3,6] (with aspirin or acetaminophen)	180-200 mg q 3-4 h	130 mg q 3-4 h
Hydrocodone[3] (Lorcet®, Lortab®, Vicodin®)	30 mg q 3-4 h	N/A
Oxycodone[3] (Percocet®, Percodan®, Roxicodone™, Tylox®)	30 mg q 3-4 h	N/A

[1]Caution: Recommended doses do not apply to patients with renal or hepatic insufficiency or other conditions affecting drug metabolism and kinetics.
[2]Caution: For morphine, hydromorphone, and oxymorphone, rectal administration is an alternate route for patients unable to take oral medications. Equianalgesic doses may differ from oral and parenteral doses because of pharmacokinetic differences. **Note:** A short-acting opioid should normally be used for initial therapy of moderate to severe pain.
[3]Transdermal fentanyl (Duragesic®) is an alternative option. See Table 6.

Usual starting dose for
moderate to severe pain

Oral	Parenteral
0.3 mg/kg q 3-4 h	0.1 mg/kg q 3-4 h
N/A	N/A
0.06 mg/kg q 3-4 h	0.015 mg/kg q 3-4 h
0.04 mg/kg q 6-8 h	0.02 mg/kg q 6-8 h
N/R	0.75 mg/kg q 2-3 h
0.2 mg/kg q 6-8 h	0.1 mg/kg q 6-8 h
0.5-1 mg/kg q 3-4 h	N/R
0.2 mg/kg q 3-4 h	N/A
0.2 mg/kg q 3-4 h	N/A

See the package insert for dosing calculations. Doses above 25 µg/h should not be used in opioid-naive patients.
[4]Not recommended. Doses listed are for brief therapy. Switch to another opioid for long-term therapy.
[5]Caution: Doses of aspirin and acetaminophen in combination opioid/NSAID preparations must also be adjusted to the patient's body weight.
[6]Caution: Some clinicians recommend not exceeding 1.5 mg/kg of codeine because of increased incidence of side effects with higher doses.

Table 4: Noninvasive Analgesia for Patients With Moderate to Severe Pain

Converting from parenteral patient-controlled morphine pumps or continuous morphine infusion to morphine sulfate tablets

Average hourly morphine dose (mg/h)	Equivalent daily oral morphine dose (mg/day)	Approximate equianalgesic q 12 h* regimen of morphine sulfate tablets
1	72	2 tablets 15 mg q 12 h
2	144	2 tablets 30 mg q 12 h
3	216	3 tablets 30 mg q 12 h
4	288	2 tablets 60 mg q 12 h
5	360	3 tablets 60 mg q 12 h
6	432	3 tablets 60 mg q 12 h
7	504	4 tablets 60 mg q 12 h
8	576	4 tablets 60 mg q 12 h
9	648	3 tablets 100 mg q 12 h
10	720	3 tablets 100 mg q 12 h
15	1,080	5 tablets 100 mg q 12 h
20	1,440	7 tablets 100 mg q 12 h
25	1,800	9 tablets 100 mg q 12 h
30	2,160	10 tablets 100 mg q 12 h
35	2,520	12 tablets 100 mg q 12 h
40	2,880	14 tablets 100 mg q 12 h

*Individual patients will differ when converted to oral morphine and may need to be titrated up or down. Be prepared to assess the patient's level of pain and the presence of side effects, and titrate as necessary. (Adapted and printed with permission of the Purdue Frederick Co., Norwalk, CT.)

Side Effects of Oral Narcotics

The most common side effects involve the gastrointestinal tract and cognition. Narcotics produce constipation and nausea in a substantial number of patients. Both must be managed. Constipation can be treated with the usual measures well known to most physicians. Nausea is a more complicated issue and may re-

> **Table 5: Alternative Procedures for Converting Patients from IV Morphine to Morphine Sulfate Tablets**
>
> 1. Calculate average hourly IV morphine dose.
>
> 2. Use chart in Table 4 to determine approximate equianalgesic regimen of morphine sulfate tablets.
>
> 3. Either: Stop the IV infusions and administer an equivalent amount of morphine sulfate tablets, and adjust dosage as necessary, or
>
>   Gradually decrease the IV infusion while increasing the oral morphine sulfate tablets. Adjust dosage as necessary.
>
>   - On day 1, reduce infusion by half and add half of the morphine sulfate tablet dose. Adjust dosage as necessary.
>
>   - On day 2, reduce infusion by half, and increase the morphine sulfate tablet dose by half of the adjusted day-1 dosage. Adjust dosage as necessary.
>
>   - On day 3, stop infusion and administer full (adjusted) dose of morphine sulfate tablets. Adjust dosage as necessary.
>
> (Adapted and printed with permission of the Purdue Frederick Co., Norwalk, CT.)

quire changing narcotics until one is found that does not produce nausea. When nausea persists, it can be treated with hydroxyzine hydrochloride (Atarax®) 10 mg with the opioids up to 3 times daily or twice a day with analgesic patches. Cisapride (Propulsid®) 10 to 20 mg t.i.d. before meals is another good choice. Metoclopramide (Reglan®) is excellent, but brain-related side effects limit its long-term use.

The effects on cognition are usually first seen in degraded mental function, lack of alertness and response to the environment, and depressed mood. Unfortunately, most require changing the narcotic or reducing the dose.

Table 6: Drug Conversion of Oral and Parenteral Narcotics to Transdermal Fentanyl

Transdermal fentanyl (μg/h)	Morphine oral mg/d	IM mg/d	Hydromorphone oral mg/d	IM mg/d
25*	45–134	8–22	5.6–17	1.2–3.4
50	135–224	23–37	17.1–28	3.5–5.6
75	225–314	38–52	28.1–39	5.7–7.9
100	315–404	53–67	39.1–51	8–10
125	405–494	68–82	51.1–62	10.1–12
150	495–584	83–97	62.1–73	12.1–15

Transdermal fentanyl (μg/h)	Oxycodone oral mg/d	IM mg/d	Levorphanol oral mg/d	IM mg/d
25*	22.5–67	12–33	3–8.9	1.6–4.4
50	67.5–112	33.1–56	9–14.9	4.5–7.4
75	112.5–157	56.1–78	15–20.9	7.5–10.4
100	157.5–202	78.1–101	21–26.9	10.5–13.4
125	202.5–247	101.1–123	27–32.9	13.5–16.4
150	247.5–292	123.1–147	33–38.9	16.5–19.4

Transdermal fentanyl (μg/h)	Meperidine oral mg/d	IM mg/d	Codeine oral mg/d	IM mg/d
25*	—	60–165	150–447	104–286
50	—	166–278	448–747	287–481
75	—	279–390	748–1047	482–676
100	—	391–503	1048–1347	677–871
125	—	504–615	1348–1647	872–1066
150	—	616–728	1648–1947	1067–1261

* Do not initiate transdermal fentanyl (Duragesic®) at greater than 25 μg/h in opioid-naive patients.

Note: A dosage conversion calculator is available from Janssen Pharmaceutica and should be used if higher doses are required.

Remember that myoclonus or sudden unexpected jerks throughout the body may occur with narcotic usage. The most serious problem is respiratory depression, which means patients,

Table 7: Characteristics of Transdermal Fentanyl

Transdermal fentanyl patch

- Fentanyl, a short-acting and highly potent agent, is absorbed into the skin, creating a depot in the upper layer. Active drug then becomes available to systemic circulation.
- The patch (Duragesic®) offers up to 72 h of analgesia; steady state is achieved in 12 to 16 h.
- Patients wearing fentanyl transdermal patches who develop fever should be monitored for opioid side effects and the patch dose should be adjusted if necessary.
- Short-acting opioids are easily added to manage breakthrough pain.*
- If local erythema occurs, the patch may be placed in different areas of the body.

* Manufacturer's prescribing information, including boxed warning, 1994.

particularly those on large doses of oral narcotics, need to be watched carefully.

Tolerance

Tolerance, which is decreased pain relief with a fixed dose of drug, occurs routinely with long-term narcotic management. However, increasing data indicate that tolerance is not as serious a deterrent to long-term narcotic use as was once believed. Nevertheless, it is a critical issue. Cancer patients with stable disease rarely escalate opioid dose independently. When they do, it is usually because of a change in the disease state and an increase in pain. Because these patients are physically dependent, change in medications must be managed carefully. One technique is to reduce by half the dose of the narcotic being used while changing from one drug to another. The change in drugs alone will often achieve good pain relief again. If that does not occur, the reduction of drug dose and then gradual escalation often restore appropriate analgesia.

Route of Administration of Narcotics for Cancer Pain

The pain therapist must understand not only the drugs and the progression of their use, but also the forms of administration that are most useful. Nonnarcotic analgesics and the opioids used for moderate pain are nearly always taken orally. When occasional pain control is required, parenteral routes (subcutaneous and intramuscular) are useful, but should not be employed when regular narcotic use is required. Transdermal application (Tables 6 and 7) is used if weaker opioids fail. Time-released adherent skin patches, which release analgesics over an extended period, are now commercially available.

When oral and transdermal techniques are not effective, and when pain is continuous enough that episodic parenteral injections are inadequate for control, then more permanent parenteral forms are available. These include:

(1) Intravenous administration through a permanent venous access. The IV techniques can use continuous infusion under computer control or repetitive administration when necessary. They are valuable for bringing severe pain under control initially and when life expectancy is not long.

(2) Epidural administration with an implanted catheter can provide general or segmental pain relief. An epidural catheter is placed in the general spinal cord region where the pain is most apparent. For short-term use, a percutaneous catheter is satisfactory. Also, implanted subcutaneous portal systems are available. Both the percutaneous technique and the implanted portal are satisfactory when life expectancy is not long. For patients expected to live for a year or more, computer-controlled implanted pumps are effective, but their major drawback is cost.

All these systems have the advantage of providing adequate analgesia in most patients while requiring very low doses of narcotics so that systemic effects are minimized. Frequently, pain control can be achieved by doses of 2.5 mg to 5.0 mg of morphine daily.

(3) Intrathecal narcotic injection is analogous to epidural injection, although it entails more difficulty in replacing the catheter. It is not generally used with a percutaneous catheter because of the risk of infection, but subcutaneous portals and implanted pumps provide excellent ways to deliver intrathecal narcotic. The drug dosage can be even smaller. The narcotic must be pyrogen-free, which is a limiting factor.

(4) Intraventricular narcotics are also a feasible way to relieve pain. The catheter must be placed percutaneously through the lateral ventricles into the posterior third ventricle. There, minute quantities of narcotic delivered into this region of the ventricular system will produce excellent pain relief without systemic side effects. The technique requires an expert at catheter placement and careful monitoring while drug doses are adjusted.

Because of the risks involved, we keep all patients undergoing intrathecal or intraventricular test injections in an intensive care unit for observation of the effect of the drug.

Surgical Management of Cancer Pain

Surgical procedures that intentionally destroy a part of the nervous system have their greatest application in the treatment of cancer pain.[4] These types of operations were used extensively until the long-acting oral narcotics were developed, making pain relief with oral agents feasible. Destructive procedures are used less often now, but they still can play an important part in cancer pain management. Some patients have pain that cannot be relieved by acceptable oral doses of analgesics. Other patients have intolerable side effects from drugs, even at low doses. Surgical procedures can permanently relieve pain and eliminate the need for narcotics that are ineffective or produce unacceptable side effects.[4,5]

General Factors

When a surgical approach is contemplated, the health-care team must be certain of the cause of the pain. Destructive procedures can be useful for pain secondary to tissue invasion or other direct effects of tumor. They are less useful in neuropathic pain. The general status of the patient is important. Also, life expectancy should be adequate to warrant the procedure, particularly if open operation is required. Percutaneous techniques can produce excellent pain control for which the patient will be grateful even if life expectancy is only a few weeks. All patients should have a trial of nonsurgical management. It is always worthwhile remembering the difference between pain and pain behavior. Finally, surgical procedures should be considered only when the clinician is certain that anxiety and depression are effectively managed.

Surgical Procedures for Pain

1. Spinal Dorsal Rhizotomy. The oldest surgical procedure for pain relief is division of the spinal nerves or roots. The technique is not very useful in the extremities because the neurologic deficit is usually unacceptable. Rhizotomy has its greatest use in the thorax and abdomen and is particularly used for chest pain secondary to wall invasion by tumor. The technique requires identification of the number of roots that must be divided to achieve pain relief. Rhizotomy may be unilateral or bilateral. Temporary blockade of the suspected painful roots can determine which roots should be divided.

The spinal rhizotomy can be done in several ways. The simplest is a percutaneous heat destructive lesion of the nerves involved in the painful process. The technique is painful and requires a general anesthetic. Radiofrequency needles are directed near the nerve in the neuroforamen and the nerve is coagulated. Several nerves on each side can easily be treated with only resultant sensory loss. The motor disturbance is not important in the thoracic region. The principal risk of the procedure is paraplegia if an important nutrient artery is coagulated. This is extremely rare.

The second technique is to simply cut the spinal nerves at the exit from the spine or at some convenient place beneath a rib. This is feasible in the thoracic region, but not elsewhere. More commonly, these operations are performed by neurosurgeons via laminectomy or hemilaminectomy. The operation is intradural and this allows the posterior roots to be cut, thus denervating the painful area. Others have also described selective division of the laterally placed pain-carrying fibers.

Rhizotomy techniques are effective when the disease is limited and when all of the pain-carrying nerves plus one above and one below can be divided. The resultant sensory loss is not critical to the average patient, but there is a risk of spinal cord injury from vascular occlusion. The technique may be used occasionally to interrupt abdominal innervation, but rhizotomy is used only for chest pain and head and neck pain, as described below.

2. Cranial Rhizotomy. Head and neck pain can be effectively treated by rhizotomy. Typically, the head and neck are denervated by division of the fifth (V) cranial nerve, the nervus intermedius, and the ninth (IX) cranial nerve with upper cervical posterior rhizotomy of C1, C2, and C3. This operation divides the sensory fibers from the face and side of the head, mouth, pharynx, and upper neck. It is used primarily for indolent neoplasms in patients whose life expectancy is long. The operation is complicated and should not be undertaken in patients who are not in good general condition. The risks are small and the denervation of the face, mouth, and throat unilaterally do not have major functional significance. These patients will have some difficulty in managing secretions on that side, but should be able to function normally. The operation is carried out by suboccipital craniectomy supplemented by upper cervical hemilaminectomy.

3. Cordotomy. Anterolateral spinal tractotomy is a successful, time-honored way to relieve cancer pain. The goal is to interrupt ascending pain fibers that make up the anterolateral spinothalamic tract. Dividing the tract results in complete loss of pain and temperature sensation on the side of the body opposite the lesion and usually in several segments below the actual area of cord injury. Cordotomy is most useful when the pain is unilateral, but bilateral cordotomies are possible. Traditionally, the cord sections are made in the thoracic region at T1-2 when the pain is in the pelvis or lower or in the midcervical (C5-6) and high cervical (C1-2) regions when the pain is above the pelvis.

Open Cervical Cordotomy. The traditional cordotomy requires general anesthesia and open operation. The spinal cord is exposed at the required location, a hemilaminectomy is performed, the dura is opened, and, under direct vision, a knife is used to cut the spinothalamic tract, which is located superficially in the anterior quadrant of the spinal cord. There is a homotopic relationship, with sacral fibers being most superficial and lateral and cervical fibers being most medial. A skilled surgeon can denervate a part of the body and leave the remainder unaffected.

Percutaneous Cervical Cordotomy. Percutaneous techniques were developed to reduce the risks of major open operation in patients who are often quite ill from their systemic disease. The percutaneous technique also makes application of cordotomy feasible in patients in poor physical condition with short life expectancy. The technique is performed under local anesthesia. A fine radiofrequency needle is passed into the spinal cord under direct fluoroscopic control from the lateral approach through the C1-2 neuroforamen. When the needle is in place in the anterior quadrant, radiofrequency current is used to coagulate the spinothalamic tract.

Results of Cordotomy. Unilateral cordotomy is effective for disease limited to one side of the body. Nearly 95% of patients achieve pain relief immediately. There is an early failure rate, but 85% to 90% of patients overall achieve good pain control with minimal risk. The major risk is injury to the corticospinal tract with a resultant contralateral hemiparesis. Bilateral procedures are less effective and the risks are higher. Patients undergoing bilateral cordotomy are more likely to develop paresis and to have difficulty walking. Still, most do not have deficits and pain relief is usually satisfactory.

Bilateral high cervical cordotomy carries a special risk. When asleep, such patients often lose their drive to breathe. This is called Ondine's curse, after the German legend, and is usually fatal.

Pain control after cordotomy usually persists for at least a year and sometimes longer. However, recurrence of pain is common with time. So, in general, cordotomy has been used for patients who are going to live more than a few months, but less than 2 years. The best results have occurred in these patients. Cordotomy is particularly useful in patients who cannot tolerate narcotics because of unpleasant cognitive side effects.

4. Commissural Myelotomy. Division of the pain-carrying crossing fibers in the anterior commissure is a highly specialized neurosurgical operation useful principally for intractable pelvic pain. The operation requires a general anesthetic. The spinal cord is exposed through full laminectomy at the level of the pain-carrying segments and above. The spinal cord is literally split down the midline so that transmission of all the crossing fibers from the painful segments is interrupted. The operation is usually done just above the conus medullaris. It is very effective for cancer pain. Patients typically have unpleasant sensations for a few days and may have transient weakness in both legs. Some gait disturbance may be permanent, but lower extremity function generally remains satisfactory. The great risk is to bowel and bladder function, but because most of these patients have advanced pelvic cancer, they already have lost bowel and bladder function before the procedure. I do not use it in patients whose bowel and bladder function remains relatively normal.

5. Cingulumotomy. Another neurosurgical operation useful for cancer pain is destruction of the cingulum, a stereotactic procedure that can be done under local anesthesia. The cingulum is localized just above the corpus callosum over the anterior lateral ventricles bilaterally. Bilateral cingulumotomy provides effective pain relief in many patients. It is particularly useful in patients with anxiety and depression that have not responded to other treatments and that seriously complicate pain management. Patients with disfiguring head and neck tumors often will respond well to cingulumotomy. There are few side effects, but some changes in cognition may occur and must be considered in making the decision.

Other techniques have been employed, but are no longer used except in unusual circumstances. The upper cervical region and head can be denervated by medullary trigeminal tractotomy. This technique was originally developed for trigeminal neuralgia and then used in cancer pain. Because it carries a substantial risk of unilateral cerebellar dysfunction, it is rarely used now. This is a procedure for a surgeon who is expert in the technique.

6. Thalamotomy has been used extensively for cancer pain. Several targets in the thalamus have been described. In general, the reported outcomes have not been good and thalamotomy has been supplanted by other techniques. Whether new physiologic and anatomical information will make thalamotomy a valuable technique for cancer pain is not yet certain.

7. Hypophysectomy has been used extensively for pain from breast and prostate cancer. The technique is most useful for advanced breast cancer where success rates have been reasonable. The outcome in prostatic cancer is less encouraging. The original operation required subfrontal craniotomy. This was supplanted by transsphenoidal hypophysectomy. Now pituitary ablation with radiofrequency or chemical means is possible. The great negative is induced pituitary insufficiency. Hypophysectomy was once a valuable adjunct in the treatment of widely disseminated breast cancer. Newer management techniques have almost eliminated the need for hypophysectomy in either prostate or breast cancer.

References

1. Foley KM: The treatment of cancer pain. *N Engl J Med* 1985; 313:84-95.

2. Payne R, Foley KM, eds: *The Medical Clinics of North America: Cancer Pain.* Philadelphia, WB Saunders Co, 1987.

3. Twycross RG: The management of pain in cancer. In: Nimmo WS, Smith G, eds. *Anaesthesia.* vol 2. Oxford, Blackwell Scientific Publications, 1988, pp 1216-1229.

4. Gybels JM, Sweet WH: *Neurosurgical Treatment of Persistent Pain.* Basel, Karger, 1989.

5. Long DM: Surgical therapy of chronic pain. *Neurosurgery* 1980; 6(3):317-328.

Chapter 5

Evaluation and Management of Low Back Pain

Low back pain, with or without leg pain, is one of the two most common pain complaints in America today, equalled only by headache. Low back pain remains the most common cause of industrial disability and of Social Security payments for physical disability. Population studies suggest that its prevalence in the adult population is at least 60% and its incidence is 30%. At any given time, 10% to 12% of the population is seeking health care for low back pain.

Characteristics of low back pain mirror those of pain in general. Low back pain tends to be temporal (related to the time the pain lasts), or based on estimates of severity. The presence or absence of referred radicular pain is another differentiating factor.

The causes of low back pain are many and varied, but degenerative disk disease (spondylosis) appears to be the underlying factor for most patients. Another large group of patients seems to have muscular and ligamentous inflammatory disease, which is poorly characterized at present. Low back pain is seen as a complication of many other problems, including cancer, infection, rheumatologic disease, and a host of rare conditions. A well-recognized factor that makes attribution of cause difficult is that changes typical of spondylosis occur without related pain. All of these factors make it difficult to classify low back pain according to etiology.[1,2]

Classification Scheme for Low Back Pain

Many low back pains cited in population studies are *transient*. Usually activity related, these pains may be severe, but typically resolve within a few hours. Patients with transient episodes rarely seek medical attention unless the frequency of the pain events becomes intolerable.

However, the typical back patient that the general physician sees suffers from *acute* low back pain. The pain has a spontaneous onset in about half the cases and trauma is usually identified by the patient in the other half. Low back pain characteristically radiates to the hips, groin, and anterior and posterior thighs. Nonradicular pain below the knees is unusual. Low back pain may be associated with typical sciatic radiation. The sciatic syndrome will be described in the section on intervertebral disk herniation.

Persistent low back pain is similar, but fails to improve and lasts more or less without change for months or years. The word *chronic* could be used just as effectively, but we have chosen persistent to typify these patients to separate them from the chronic pain syndrome in which personality dysfunction and psychosocial and medical comorbidities are common (see Chapter 14).

Common Diagnostic Labels Encountered in Low Back Pain

(1) *Lumbosacral strain or sprain.* This implies a muscular and ligamentous injury similar to an ankle sprain.

(2) *Disk herniation.* This diagnosis should be made only when the nucleus pulposus has been displaced from the intervertebral space and now lies in the spinal canal or foramen or outside the foramen. A loose cartilage fragment is called a free fragment. A bulging disk indicates that the fragment is still contained by the longitudinal ligament or that the nucleus has herniated diffusely without fragmenting. A degenerated disk indicates that there is no herniation, but that the entire nucleus, and perhaps the annulus, has undergone drying and degeneration.

(3) *Diskogenic syndrome.* This imprecise term suggests that the pain is coming from the lumbar disk. Those who believe it exists indicate tears in the annulus, release of chemical mediators, or micromotion as the generators of pain.

(4) *Spondylolysis.* This indicates a structural defect in the pars interarticularis.

(5) *Spondylolisthesis.* This term describes slipping of one vertebral segment on another. The slip may be forward or backward, in which case it is called retrolisthesis.

(6) *Facet syndrome.* Speculation for many years has suggested that much unexplained back pain originates in the facets, which are better called zygapophyseal joints. This pain is located only in the back, is aggravated by movement (particularly by rotation), and is improved by rest. So-called facet blocks anesthetize the facets to determine if they play a role in pain. Percutaneous denervation has been advocated for this syndrome.

(7) *Spondylosis.* This general term describes all of the changes that occur with degenerative disk disease, including desiccation of the disk, narrowing of the interspace, inflammatory and degenerative changes in the bone, ligament hypertrophy, and bony spurring.

(8) *Spinal stenosis.* This is used to describe the condition in which the spinal canal is narrowed either congenitally or from spondylosis. The narrowing may be of the whole canal, in the lateral recess, or isolated to the neural foramina.

(9) *Spinal instability.* This can be a difficult concept to understand because of the controversy that exists about the definition of instability. The simplest way to explain this is that the spine is unstable when movement of bony elements is identified on flexion/extension or on motion films. Progressive slipping of the spine, as documented on repeated studies, is another way to make the diagnosis. When the abnormality is not extreme, the arguments begin. Some believe in the concept of micromotion, that is, movement that cannot be identified with any of our current tests, but which produces pain. Much argument among experts concerns what constitutes adequate evidence for spinal instability. Until better definitions are available, the term should be reserved for the obvious movement of the spine with motion or over time.

(10) *Failed back syndrome.* This term is used to denote patients who have undergone more than one spinal surgery and

still have incapacitating complaints. It is imprecise and only describes the failure of surgical treatment.[3,4]

Functional Anatomy of the Lumbar Spine

Normally, there are five lumbar spinal segments, and the sacrum is a part of the functional unit. These five vertebral bodies are similar in shape and their disks and ligamentous structures are similar, but they are not exactly the same. The heaviest portion of the bone is located anteriorly and termed the vertebral body. Between these bodies lie the intervertebral disks. On the anterior surface of the body is a very strong ligament, the anterior longitudinal ligament. On the posterior surface of the body within the spinal canal is an equally strong posterior longitudinal ligament. The intervertebral disk is composed of two parts. The annulus fibrosis is a heavy circle of thick collagen that contains the soft compressible nucleus pulposus. The annulus binds tightly to the surrounding bodies, inserting into the periosteum and incorporating the longitudinal ligaments. The spinal canal is posterior to the bodies and bound laterally by bony struts called pedicles and posteriorly by the laminae. The exit areas for spinal nerves are called foramina. Posteriorly, the zygapophyseal joints (facets) are the articulating joints between successive vertebrae. These are true cartilaginous joints. The bony anatomy is completed by a midline spine that extends posteriorly and by the lateral extensions called transverse processes. These are bound together by heavy ligaments and serve as sites of attachment for the major muscles. Heavy paravertebral muscles are located posteriorly, inserting on spinous processes, laminae, lateral structures, and transverse processes. These are bound together in the midline by the lumbar fascia. Similar anterior longitudinal muscles are attached to the transverse processes and to anterolateral portions of the vertebral bodies.

A single body with its attached disk, ligaments, and joints is called a motion segment. The motion segment includes parts of two bodies, a disk, and the joints articulating the posterior elements at that level. Thus, a motion segment is often described as L4-5, which denotes the structures that relate L4 to L5. All the lumbar segments are described this way.

Many of these structures are capable of generating pain. Pain receptors are found in the ligaments, the muscle, on the periosteum, and in the annulus fibrosis. They are probably present in the cartilage of joints, and certainly in the ligaments binding zygapophyseal joints together.

Painful Pathologic Changes in the Lumbosacral Spine

(1) *Disk degeneration.* Simple degeneration of a lumbar disk may cause pain, but disk degeneration without pain is common. We cannot now define painful disk degeneration by any certain imaging criteria. Therefore, the simple fact that degeneration occurs will not necessarily explain a pain problem. Nevertheless, the incidence of spondylitic change in patients complaining of back pain is so common that most experts agree the two are related in ways that are not now understood.

(2) *Disk herniation.* Disk herniation is when the nucleus pulposus partly or completely herniates through a defect in the annulus. The typical herniation occurs into the lateral spinal canal at the level of the disk. Migration of a free fragment can occur. Disk herniations also occur into the neural foramina and may occur laterally or anteriorly as well. Most patients with true disk herniation have symptoms that suggest nerve root irritation. That is, the pain radiates in the anatomic distribution of the nerve being compressed.

(3) *Joint arthritis.* Most experts now agree that degenerative changes of the zygapophyseal joints can cause pain. There is still much debate about treatment, but with MRI it is now possible to identify these arthritic changes. What role the abnormalities play in an individual patient is often difficult to determine. Patients characteristically have back pain with radiation to hips and groin as well as to anterior or posterior thighs. Rotational movements are particularly painful. Rest helps, as does bracing. Anesthetization of the zygapophyseal joints should relieve the pain completely. Percutaneous denervation of the joints and posterolateral fusion are both recommended treatments.

(4) *Spinal stenosis.* Patients with spinal stenosis often complain of nondescript back pain. However, the typical abnormali-

ty is neurogenic claudication; that is, when a patient walks, his or her legs become progressively painful and progressively dysfunctional. It may be indistinguishable from vascular claudication, hence the name. Typically, however, vascular claudication symptoms disappear quickly with rest while so-called neurogenic claudication requires several minutes and often an acutely flexed position to achieve relief of symptoms. Neurologic findings often suggest peripheral neuropathy with a stocking sensory loss being present or accompanying the claudication.

(5) *Foraminal stenosis.* Spinal stenosis can occur in the foramen. The exit for the nerve is reduced in diameter and the nerve is apparently compressed by bone in the foramen. Symptoms can be indistinguishable from the herniated disk. Typically, pain occurs in the distribution of the nerve being compressed, and sensory, motor, and reflex changes should suggest the nerve involved.

(6) *Spondylolysis and spondylolisthesis.* These patients have a defect in the pars interarticularis that causes back pain. Leg pain will occur only if the movement compresses a nerve root. Pain is usually worsened by movement and improved by rest, but has no other special characteristic.

(7) *Scoliosis.* With degenerative change the spine may become scoliotic. Displacements may be rotational or there may be simple curves that deform the spine. The spine may become excessively straight (flat back syndrome) or angled anteriorly (kyphosis). All of these structural abnormalities produce back pain, but no specific syndromes.

Causes of Low Back Pain

Acute low back pain is most commonly muscular or ligamentous in origin. Some acute low back syndromes apparently originate from injury to zygapophyseal joints. Others suggest that minor annular tears cause these acute back syndromes. A truly herniated disk may present with acute back and leg pain. When the herniation is associated with nerve root compression, sciatica is common.

Recurrent low back pain has the same general causes. Patients are more likely to show evidence of degenerative disk disease and facet arthropathy. Root compression syndromes may be caused by foraminal compression or chronic disk herniation, but pain need not be constant. The typical patient coming to surgery for lumbar herniated disk has a history of years of recurrent episodes of acute low back pain before the final disk herniation occurs. Some evidence suggests that the disk slowly works its way through a weakened annulus before the final herniation occurs. Chronic low back pain is most commonly associated with significant degenerative disk disease, facet arthropathy, and/or evidence of lumbar instability.

It is always worth remembering that low back syndromes can be caused by diseases other than lumbar spondylosis. Bony fracture, ligamentous disruption of a joint, or annular tear may be the precipitating cause of pain when there is a history of trauma. Rarely, a serious systemic disease such as metastatic neoplasm will be found. Spontaneous disk space infection is even more rare. True disk herniation is actually a rare cause of back and leg pain. Typical population studies suggest that no more than 2% of people complaining of significant back pain will harbor a herniated disk. Retroperitoneal disease may mimic lumbar spondylosis. Spontaneous back pain complicates diabetes and acromegaly and occurs in both rheumatoid and ankylosing spondylitis as well as even rarer rheumatologic diseases.

History and Physical Examination in Low Back Pain

The history is the most important aspect of the examination. The physical findings will be diagnostic only with the truly herniated disk and even then may be nonspecific. The first issue is the severity of the pain because the extent of the investigation and the therapy will depend on how serious the pain is. Most low back attacks, even those that are severe, are not characterized by excruciating pain. When the pain is severe, the clinician should consider fracture, metastatic disease, or infection. The location of the pain is also important. If the pain is in the lumbar region without sciatic radiation, then it is unlikely that substantial nerve root compression has occurred. Nonspecific radiation to the buttocks, hips, groins, and anterior or posterior thighs can occur in any low back pain syndrome; these radiations do not suggest nerve root compression. Herniations at the L4-5 and L5-S1 spaces typically produce sciatica, and the pain follows the course of the sciatic nerve posteriorly. When L5 is involved, the pain goes to the top of the foot and the great toe. When S1 is involved, pain occurs at the lateral side of the foot and the sole. Pain from upper disk herniation at L1-2, L2-3, or L3-4 typically follows the course of the femoral nerve on the anterior thigh and may be difficult to differentiate from nonspecific anterior thigh radiation. Most pain that is secondary to lumbar spondylosis is alleviated by rest and aggravated by activity. It fluctuates according to the patient's activity level. Pain that is constant and unchanged by activity suggests tumor or infection. Night pain particularly suggests tumor. Significant neurologic complaints such as weakness, numbness, sciatic pain, or abnormalities of bowel and bladder function always suggest neurologic involvement.

Physical examination begins with inspection of the back. The spine should be straight and there should be a slight lordotic curve. Palpation will reveal the presence or absence of paravertebral muscle spasm. Scoliosis new in onset suggests asymmetric spasm more severe on the concave side. Muscle spasm frequently elevates one hip and the obvious pelvic asymmetry frequently concerns patients. This functional change is often misinterpreted as a short extremity. Examine range of motion. Patients should be able to flex, extend, and rotate without pain. Some believe that rotational movements suggest facet disease, but in the experience of most clinicians, all of these changes are nonspecific and only indicate the presence or absence of local muscle changes. The examination should include assessment of gait if possible, looking for weakness. Examine the strength of all muscle groups. Examine sensation in the lower extremities to pin prick and light touch. Position sense and vibration sense can be assessed, but are rarely useful unless a polyneuropathy is suspected. Sciatic and femoral tension signs are important. Straight leg raising can be done with the patient seated or supine. The straight leg is lifted and the angle at which the typical radiating sciatic pain is produced is recorded. For the test to be positive, sciatica must be reproduced. The presence of back pain only is nonspecific. A crossed straight leg raising is positive when the nonpainful leg lift causes the contralateral pain to occur. The femoral nerve is stretched by extending the hip, and this maneuver should cause pain. Rarely, hip joint disease can mimic sciatica from nerve root compression, so the Patrick's maneuver for hip joint disease can be done as well.

The actual examination can be simple. My routine is as follows: I examine the back, palpate the paravertebral muscles, and have the patient extend, flex, and rotate. The patient is asked to stand and walk so the gait can be observed. Then the patient is balanced by the examiner and is asked to stand on toes and on heels. Weakness of plantar flexion and dorsiflexion are thus easily seen. The knee and ankle reflexes are checked, then the patient is asked about sensation. If a patient can walk in the dark without a light, proprioception is intact. If the patient does not experience sensory loss or sensory aberrations, then it is unlikely that any sensory changes exist. Any perceived sensory loss is then checked with light touch and pin prick and verified. The physical examination typically takes no more than 5 minutes.

The legs are also inspected for asymmetry. Measurement may be necessary to document minor degrees of asymmetry, but these are of questionable importance. The appearance of the skin is examined and lower extremity pulse is determined.

Herniated Lumbar Disk Syndrome

Lumbar disk herniation with individual root compression produces specific syndromes that are well localized by the description of the pain and the physical examination.

Disk herniation at L5-S1 may affect either the L5 or the S1 disk. S1 involvement is characterized by sciatic pain, an absent ankle reflex, weakness of plantar flexion, and sensory loss in the lateral third of the foot and the sole. L5 involvement is signalled by sciatic radiation, weakness of dorsiflexion of the foot and toes, and sensory loss on the dorsum of the foot, particularly involving the great toe. L4-5 disk herniation may affect L4 or L5. The L4 syndrome is characterized by pain radiating in the distribution of the femoral nerve, often to just below the knee. The patellar reflex is reduced and sensory loss occurs around the knee and on the anterolateral leg. Quadriceps weakness results in weak leg extension. Straight leg raising will be positive with disk herniations in either location. Disk herniation in the three upper lumbar spaces is rare. Sensory loss and motor weakness will occur in the anterior thigh. There are no reflex changes. Femoral stretch by leg extension will reproduce the pain.

Spinal Stenosis Syndrome or Neurogenic Claudication

Stenosis of the spinal canal produces neurogenic claudication, a syndrome that may be hard to differentiate from vascular claudication. Such patients will have back and leg pain that increases with walking, and leg weakness that ensues with walking. The legs become numb and weak because a stocking hypesthesia develops. The syndrome is frequently thought to be psychosomatic in origin. It may be confused with metabolic polyneuropathy. A factor differentiating it from vascular claudication is the duration of symptoms. Typically, the patient with vascular claudication has diminished peripheral pulses and prompt resolution of symptoms as soon as activity stops. The patient with neurogenic claudication typically has preserved pulses in the lower extremities. Symptoms are relieved by flexion of the spine, but require several minutes or more to relent. As the syndrome progresses, the neurologic deficit becomes fixed and a true cauda equina syndrome may develop. This includes weakness in both lower extremities, stocking hypesthesia concordant with the level of stenosis, and diminished bowel, bladder, and sexual function.

Imaging Studies of the Lumbar Spine

The new imaging studies provide a detailed assessment of the anatomy of the lumbar spine, but often they cannot demonstrate the cause of pain. Determining the exact cause of pain for most people with low back pain with and without sciatica is still a major diagnostic challenge.

Most experts begin with plain lumbosacral spine films. These should include AP, lateral, and oblique views and flexion/extension. The bony anatomy is well seen, but soft tissues are not. The arthritic changes of lumbar spondylosis and degenerative disk disease will be seen well. The plain films may demonstrate an unexpected tumor, trauma, or congenital anomalies. Occasionally, related paravertebral disease is identified, but definitive diagnosis generally requires further study.

The MRI has replaced virtually all other studies for examination of the spine. Computerized axial tomography (CAT) still has value, but it is generally less useful than MRI, which demonstrates soft tissues well. MRI can define disk herniation with great accuracy and assess most other soft tissue diseases. However, bony anatomy is not well seen. CAT scan is better for bone imaging. The two can be used in conjunction, but for most patients MRI is the procedure of choice and the only imaging technique required. Specialized studies, such as three-dimensional CT and CT-myelography, are reserved for specific diagnostic problems and are most useful in the failed back syndrome. When to have these studies is very important. Most experts agree that acute back pain does not require imaging unless the pain does not relent spontaneously. Most advise no imaging studies for at least the first month unless the pain is severe, or there is something unusual about the character, or other systemic disease or injury are suspected. When the pain has persisted for 1 to 3 months, imaging with plain films and MRI is reasonable. Remember that changes with spondylosis, that is, degenerative disk disease and facet arthropathy, occur in close to half the population, many of whom will be asymptomatic. Simply finding evidence of disk disease does not explain the low back pain syndrome. It is also important to remember that movements of 2 mm to 3 mm are normal and up to 4 or 5 may be.

Clinicians should also remember that simply finding evidence of minor movement (2 mm to 4 mm) or the presence of degenerative disk disease does not prove a symptomatic spinal abnormality.

Guidelines for Management of Acute Back Pain

The Agency for Health Policy has recently published guidelines for the management of acute back pain that most experts endorse, with individual modifications. Therefore, the interpretation of these guidelines is idiosyncratic and other experts will disagree. This is the program I use and these are the reasons why I do what I do.

Should the Patient Have an Imaging Study?

The first issue is whether a patient suffering from an acute low back syndrome for no more than a few days should be imaged. In general, the answer is no. However, if there is a history of trauma, then it is reasonable to proceed with imaging immediately. If the pain is unusually severe, recalcitrant to treatment, constant without alleviation, particularly bad at night, or associated with symptoms of systemic disease or a history of neoplasia, then immediate imaging is reasonable. This decision must be made by the individual physician and depends on the patient's complaints. The presence of significant neurologic deficit is a good reason to proceed.

What Treatments Are Useful?

Most agree that short periods of rest are worthwhile. Evidence suggests that patients actually benefit by returning to activity as soon as it is tolerated. Prolonged rest is not indicated. Rest of a few days is reasonable, but more than 1 week is virtually never indicated.

What Analgesics Are Useful?

If return to function is a goal, then providing analgesia is important. Muscle relaxants may be useful although improvement is usually marginal. I rarely use them for more than 2 weeks of an acute episode. It is more important to provide adequate analgesia. If nonnarcotic analgesics suffice, they should be used, as can the entire spectrum of nonsteroidal preparations. If a few doses of nonsteroidal medication are not satisfactory, I move immediately to oral narcotics such as codeine (Empirin® with Codeine, Tylenol® with Codeine), 30 mg to 60 mg, or oxycodone (Percodan®, Roxicet™, Tylox®), 5 mg to 10 mg. Narcotics should not be required for more than a few days. My own rule is no more than 1 week without reassessment. I do not use parenteral drugs.

Typically, prescribing bed rest for a few days with muscle relaxants and analgesics for comfort is effective. Most of these events last no longer than 1 week. Some patients find hot or cold applications to the back increase comfort.

Should the Patient Have Physical Therapy?

There is little or no evidence that passive physical therapies such as heat, massage, or ultrasound provide more than temporary improvement. Controlled trials of manipulation therapy, epidural steroid injection, and acupuncture demonstrate little or no clinically important effect on the acute low back pain syndrome. Therefore, I do not use any of these techniques. There is no evidence that bracing is warranted in the acute phase. The data suggest that transcutaneous electrical nerve stimulation (TENS) provides added analgesia during application, but does not shorten the duration of the pain.

It is also worthwhile exploring what the patient does that aggravates the back pain. Modifications in personal or vocational function might reduce the incidence of these attacks. Weight control is rational, although it is not proven that weight reduction changes the natural history of back pain attacks. There is reasonable evidence that an exercise program designed to strengthen axial musculature will reduce the incidence and severity of acute back pain. When the patient has fully recovered, it is reasonable to begin such a program even though the evidence is marginal that educational programs and exercise modify the natural history of this disease.

What About Traction?

Pelvic or leg traction used to be a staple in the treatment of low back pain, often for several weeks. For the most part, gravity traction has replaced pelvic traction. I do not believe these active techniques are useful in acute low back pain.

Most acute low back pain with or without sciatica or acute disk herniation is a benign, self-limited process that will disappear within 1 month. Some episodes linger longer, but nearly all will disappear within 3 months. Most patients are not incapacitated for more than a week or two. The evidence is minimal that any of the popular therapies significantly alters the natural history of this disease. My approach to these patients is a short period of rest, adequate analgesia, restoration to function as soon as possible, and then an exercise program designed to minimize recurrence.

The Persistent Low Back Syndrome

Some patients do not recover within 3 months. These patients have been neglected in most taxonomies of pain and their natural history has not been differentiated from the general acute low back pain population until recently. If back and/or leg pain persists for 3 to 6 months after onset, spontaneous improvement generally does not occur. These patients are significantly impaired by their disease. Pain persists for years, although it may vary in intensity. There is little evidence that any currently available therapies benefit these patients unless they are candidates for surgical intervention.

Diagnosis of the Persistent Pain Syndrome

Once pain has persisted for 3 months or more, complete evaluation of the patient is necessary. This should include a thorough examination for the cause of the pain and may require an expert in back pain. Plain films are important, but simply finding degenerative changes does not necessarily explain the pain. Many patients with degenerative spinal changes are asymptomatic. MRI is the best and most comprehensive examination, if only one is to be used. CT scan may be required to help guide a surgical procedure. If the pathology is expected to be bony, then CT is the best choice. Electromyography is of little use unless a peripheral neuropathy is expected. Other recommended tests, such as thermography, have not proven to be specific enough to be useful.[4]

Causes of Persistent Back Pain

The causes of unrelenting back pain are found in three broad categories. In our studies, approximately 60% of these patients have concomitant degenerative changes, that is, lumbar spondylosis. These include degenerative disk disease and spurring with nerve root compression, instability, degenerative facet joint disease, disk herniation in its various forms, and spinal stenosis.

The second cause is myofascial pain. Approximately 20% of patients in our studies are diagnosed with myofascial syndrome.

The third category is general and includes everything else. Examples are rheumatoid arthritis and the other generalized or specific spinal arthropathies, unexpected disease such as metastatic cancer, back pain complicating a systemic disease such as diabetes, congenital anomalies, spinal tumors, and, rarely, abdominal or pelvic disease, particularly retroperitoneal processes. Serious unsuspected disease accounts for less than 1% of all these patients, so urgent diagnosis is not critical.

Treatment of Persistent Back Pain

Since most low back pain patients have spondylotic disease its treatment is important. The principles are straightforward. First, be sure that the patient's complaints fit with the observed abnormalities. Simply demonstrating degenerative disk disease is not enough. If surgical therapy is to be undertaken, then root compression is an important consideration. To proceed with fusion, instability must be demonstrated. Surgery is indicated for specific reasons, described in greater detail later in this chapter. In our studies, no more than 25% of patients with spondylotic problems are candidates for surgery. Therefore, most of these patients require other forms of treatment. The national study we recently completed is instructive about these patients. First, there was no evidence that these patients improve with time. If anything, they tended to worsen slightly, but essentially stayed the same over many years.

Unfortunately, there was no indication that any of the commonly employed conservative measures changed the natural history of the disease. Standard physical therapy, including heat, massage, ultrasound, and exercise, often coupled with traction and bracing, was not beneficial. Some patients, particularly those with demonstrated instability, get some symptomatic relief with bracing. Braces also serve to protect patients by reminding them not to do things that might further stress the back. Manipulation therapy was not beneficial in these patients.

As might be expected, the number of pain management procedures offered to this frustrated group of patients beyond common physical therapy and manipulation treatments is enormous. Treatments include such diverse therapies as acupuncture, the low back school, biofeedback and cognitive treatments, psychiatric therapy, nutritional techniques, and a variety of more exotic physical therapy modes. None could be demonstrated to benefit our patients. Therefore, I conclude that none of these techniques is useful for the patient with persistent pain syndrome and therefore has no place in the treatment of low back pain and sciatica.

What Does Work?

Reasonable evidence indicates that intensive exercise programs will benefit these patients. Other programs include weight loss, although weight loss alone will not improve most patients; general physical conditioning; local measures to eliminate myofascial pain; and specific exercises for back and abdominal muscles. The exercise program appears to have the greatest long-term value and experimental evidence suggests that improvement in pathology in all the structures of the spine occurs with exercise. Most patients who enter such a specific program improve in function, although pain relief is less certain.

Myofascial Syndrome

Some patients suffer from back pain that radiates nonspecifically to hips, buttocks, groin, and upper thighs. Not only is the pain generalized, but the hallmark of the disease is the discovery of specific painful areas of inflammation in the muscles called trigger points. These trigger points are thought to be either primary or secondary to the prolonged muscle spasm. Their etiology is unknown. They are extremely painful and generate a secondary muscle spasm. In the low back they typically are in the large paravertebral muscles or the glutei. They occur in the large muscles of the thigh, but are much less common there. Trigger points are often associated with a reactive bursitis. The most common location in the lower extremities is over the greater trochanter.

Myofascial syndromes may be primary or secondary. The primary syndrome arises without related spinal disease, the secondary syndrome appears to occur when there is substantial lumbar spondylosis. They are differentiated from bursitis because they occur in muscle unrelated to bursae. Their differentiation from arthritis is not difficult because they are unrelated to joints. It is more likely that they will be confused with tendinitis, which is pain secondary to inflammation of tendinous insertions upon bone. The anatomical differences should be adequate to separate myositis from tendinitis. In the former, the problem is in the belly of the muscle. In the latter, it is at the insertion of the muscle upon bone. Acute muscle tears from trauma create a trigger point indistinguishable from the primary process, but the history of trauma usually makes the diagnosis.

Evaluation and Treatment of Myofascial Pain

The most important aspect of the evaluation is the history. Myofascial pain syndromes are reasonably specific. The pain begins in the muscles. Patients can usually show exactly where it hurts. The problem is markedly exacerbated by movement and improved by rest. Local measures such as heat and massage are often helpful. There is no radicular component. When radiation occurs, it usually does so along the plane of the muscle where the trigger point is found. Nonspecific radiation to hips, groin, and thighs is common in the low back, but does not suggest nerve root compression.

The involved muscles can be palpated and the trigger points can frequently be found by deep palpation. They are often felt as small, hard knots in the muscle that are exquisitely painful. Range of motion is impaired and movement is painful. Muscle strength may be impaired secondary to pain or disuse, but the demonstration of muscle weakness is not an important diagnostic criterion.

Imaging studies are not useful except to exclude other diseases. There is no need to image the spine with an obvious syndrome. Imaging should be reserved for those patients who do not have typical myofascial pain.

The diagnosis of myofascial pain is confirmed when trigger point injection relieves the pain. The technique is simple, with a needle at the trigger point injecting a small amount of local anesthetic. The pain from that trigger point should be promptly relieved concordant with the duration of action of the anesthetic agent. Once the diagnosis is made, direct treatments include injection of a long-acting corticosteroid, such as methylprednisolone acetate (Depo-Medrol®) 10 mg to 20 mg. If there are multiple trigger points to inject, divide 40 mg of the corticosteroid into equal doses and inject no more than that total into the trigger points. Corticosteroid injections can be repeated in 3 to 4 weeks. Be careful not to repeat so often as to produce hypercortisolism.

Repeated injection with local anesthetic over several days or weeks is also effective. Massage and TENS are also useful ways to eliminate trigger points.

Once the trigger points are under symptomatic control, either short-term from an injection or long-term from repeated therapies, it is important to begin an exercise program. The key ingredients to preventing recurrence of the trigger points are strengthening the involved muscles and restoring general physical activity.

For many patients with generalized complaints of painful muscles, a course of anti-inflammatory drugs is helpful, although no single one is specific to the pain. The choice of drugs is based on personal preference and what the patient may have used successfully before.

Surgical Intervention for Low Back Pain and Sciatica

The important principal when considering surgery for low back and leg pain is that surgery can only treat nerve root compression and spinal instability. Pain alone is never an indication for surgery. On the other hand, pain related to a correctable anatomic abnormality is the usual reason for surgery. This means that to choose a patient for surgery, the surgeon must demonstrate an anatomic abnormality that compresses a nerve root or roots or find an unstable segment of the spine. Because pain is the presenting symptom in virtually all of these patients, the uncritical surgeon can find nonspecific degenerative changes in the spine and so subject patients to operations that have little chance of success. Knowing how to choose the patient for surgery is one key to a successful outcome.

While pain is the most common reason for surgery, important neurologic deficits do occur and constitute a more obvious reason for immediate surgery. The typical syndromes are the herniated intervertebral disk, spinal stenosis, spondylolysis, and spondylolisthesis.

Surgery for the Lumbar Disk Herniation

The herniated disk is the most common reason for surgery. Patients with lumbar disk herniation usually present with acute sciatica, which is pain radiating from the low back down the course of the sciatic nerve in the distribution of the nerve root being affected. About 85% of disk herniations occur at L4-5 or L5-S1, while those that occur above usually affect the femoral nerve and radiate to the anterior thigh. The specific syndromes are:

(1) L5-S1 herniation. Disk herniation at this level usually affects either the L5 or the S1 nerve root. Pain is in the sciatic distribution. If L5 is involved, the pain radiates to the dorsum of the foot and the great toe. If S1 is involved, pain radiates to the lateral side of the foot and the sole. The L5 motor deficit is in dorsiflexion of the foot and toes. There is no associated reflex change. S1 motor deficit is in plantar flexion and the ankle reflex is generally reduced.

(2) Herniations at L4-5 may compress either the L4 or the L5 nerve root. If the L4 nerve root is compressed, then pain usually radiates in the anterior thigh to the knee and just below it. The patellar reflex is reduced and there is weakness of extension at the knee.

(3) Herniation at the L3-4 space compresses either the L3 or the L4 nerve. If the L3 nerve is involved, pain will radiate to the anterior thigh, but not below the knee. The patellar reflex may be reduced, but usually is not, and there is an associated sensory loss to approximately mid-thigh anteriorly.

(4) Higher herniations at L2-3 and L1-2 are rare. The motor deficit will be weakness of muscles of the anterior thigh and sensory loss in the upper thigh and groin. Pain radiates to mid-thigh but usually not below.

For the examination to determine these findings, begin with the patient seated, unless the pain is severe, in which case carry out the examination with the patient reclining. Check the patellar and Achilles reflexes first. Then ask the patient to stand, and examine and palpate the back. Unfortunately, signs such as muscle spasm and lack of range of motion are nonspecific and do not even occur in most patients with acute disk herniation. Nevertheless, their presence or absence should be recorded because this will make some difference in the treatment. Range of motion is examined by having the patient bend forward, bend backward, and rotate at the hips to see what degree of motion can be accomplished without pain. Trigger points can be found during palpation.

Then help balance the patient, usually just by holding the patient's hands, and ask him or her to stand successively on toes and heels. If the patient can stand on the toes symmetrically, S1 is intact. If the patient can stand on heels and symmetrical dorsiflexion is observed in both feet and toes, L5 is intact. Next, ask the patient to carry out a knee bend, again while balancing the patient. If the patient can knee bend symmetrically, the muscles of the thigh are appropriately innervated and no motor deficits are present.

If there is any question about these findings, test the muscle groups individually with the patient seated. This testing includes plantar flexion, which is pushing the foot down against resistance; dorsiflexion, which is bringing the foot and toes up against resistance; extension at the knee against resistance; flexion at the knee against resistance; and flexion at the hip against resistance. These maneuvers test all muscle groups.

Then carry out the sensory examination. Most patients will tell you the specific locations of sensory abnormalities. In fact, the patient's history of sensory abnormality is usually more accurate than the pin prick and light touch testing that we do routinely. The expected sensory abnormalities are S1—lateral two or three toes, side of foot, and sole; L5—base of great toe, great toe, dorsum, and medial foot; L4—distal anterior thigh and lateral leg just below the knee; L3—mid-thigh; and L1-2—upper thigh. Pin prick and light touch are adequate.

Then conduct the nerve stretch tests. I leave these for last because they may be very painful. Straight leg raising is done with the patient supine. The painful leg is elevated until the typical pain the patient suffers is reproduced. The production of back pain alone is a nonspecific sign that does not have localizing value. Raising the leg should reproduce the sciatic pain to be called positive. Then raise the opposite leg. If this reproduces the patient's pain, it is called the *crossed straight leg raising test* and is virtually pathognomonic for acute disk herniation. It occurs in almost no other condition. Femoral stretch is done by pulling the leg back as far as it will go, thus extending at the hip. This stretches the femoral nerve and causes pain in its distribution. It has the same significance as the straight leg raising. Straight leg raising can also be carried out with the patient seated by simply extending at the knee that stretches the nerve and causes the pain. The test is less useful than when it is done reclining. Femoral stretch can be carried out with the patient standing, but not sitting.

Many patients will have nonanatomic complaints and findings. Watch for the patient whose sensory complaints do not fit any of the patterns just given. Often patients exert little effort on motor testing. A patient who walks into the room without a limp may have an apparently paralyzed foot on specific motor testing. These are signs of an exaggerated pain syndrome, but they have no useful anatomic localization. While conducting the examination, observe the patient. Some patients will moan and groan excessively, describe pains that have no possible physiologic basis, nearly fall, and complain that the examination has excruciatingly exacerbated the pain. These reactions are known as Waddell signs and suggest either willful exaggeration or psychological vulnerability.

This basic examination requires no more than 5 minutes to complete and is usually accurately diagnostic of nerve root compression. Experts in spinal disease use imaging studies for confirmation, having made the diagnosis accurately in most patients on the basis of history and physical examination alone.

Spinal Stenosis

Spinal stenosis is usually quite different from disk herniation unless the stenosis is isolated to a single foramina with involvement of a single nerve root, which presents identically with disk herniation. The typical syndrome of spinal stenosis is called *neurogenic claudication*. Patients complain of increasing leg pain, symmetrical numbness, and symmetrical weakness with walking. It is similar to the syndrome of vascular claudication. The difference is in the recovery after cessation of activity. Patients suffering vascular claudication usually recover immediately when activity stops. Patients with neurogenic claudication typically lean forward and require several minutes or more before symptoms improve. The leaning forward opens the spinal canal and relieves the compression.

The etiology of spinal stenosis is bony and ligamentous overgrowth, sometimes associated with a congenitally small canal, causing nerve root compression in the canal. Sometimes the compression is only laterally in that portion of the canal called the lateral recess and sometimes the compression may only be in the neural foramen with lateral recess stenosis. Or foraminal stenosis compression of one or more roots is possible, so the syndrome may mimic a disk herniation. The diagnosis is made on imaging. MRI is usually adequate, but in questionable cases CT or CT-myelogram to determine bony abnormalities and relationships of bones to nerve is more accurate. The three-dimensional CT scan can be invaluable to define foraminal stenosis.

Instability Syndromes

Three fundamental abnormalities make up spinal instability. The first is spondylolysis, which denotes a specific abnormality. A bilateral defect develops in the pars interarticularis. No displacement occurs. This is a false joint that is notoriously painful. The second, spondylolisthesis, is an actual slip of the spine, either forward or back. The most typical is forward. The slip may occur because of spondylolysis or it may occur with facet joint disease. The important clinical point is that the spine is unstable. The third abnormality of the instability process is arthropathy of the zygapophyseal or facet joint. Facet arthropathy is no different from degenerative arthritis in any other cartilage joint. Degeneration of the joints and laxity of the ligaments may allow the spine to slip without a pars defect.

The clinical syndromes associated with these instability problems are much less specific than when nerve root compression has occurred. In general, the hallmark is back pain, usually worsened by activity and improved by rest. Unless nerve root compression accompanies a slip in the spine, there are no neurologic findings and the diagnoses are made by imaging studies.

The most controversial aspect of back pain is *the concept of the dysfunctional segment,* also called micromovement of the spine or simply degenerative disk disease. The problem is that many patients complain of chronic back and leg pain without any evidence of measurable instability or nerve root compression. To explain these complaints and relate them to the degenerative disk disease that is often present, the concept of the dysfunctional segment has arisen. This theory suggests that the degenerative disk itself and the changes that occur with it are the generators of the pain. Some believe the cause of the pain is chemical from materials elaborated by the degenerating disk. Some think it is mechanical and the pain is generated from the ligaments, joints, and periosteum surrounding the degenerating disk that no longer serves its support purpose. Some believe most of the pain comes from the degenerated facet joint. All of these remain theories. The treatments aimed at the dysfunctional segment are examined later in this chapter.

Indications for Intervention

Few patients are candidates for surgery.[5,6] While surgery may be beneficial when nerve root compression and/or instability is demonstrated, merely finding these abnormalities is not enough to warrant surgery or any other intervention. The first issue must be whether the patient's symptoms are serious enough to warrant a procedure. Then the time course of the disease and the presence or absence of neurologic symptoms help determine what should be done. If the patient has a significant neurologic deficit—and particularly if any bowel, bladder, or sexual dysfunction has occurred—then immediate evaluation and surgery are indicated if a correctable cause is found. Some will argue that surgery does not benefit the neurologic deficit, but that is not true in my experience. Most patients can at least be stabilized and many improved with urgent surgery. A significant neurologic deficit does not mean minor degrees of numbness and a diminished reflex. Motor dysfunction or abnormalities of bowel and bladder function are principal indications for urgent surgery, and so is intractable pain, especially in patients who cannot achieve pain relief even with heavy doses of narcotic.

When unbearable pain or significant neurologic deficit are not present, the important factor is how long the patient has had the pain. Most acute disk herniations relent, and patients will be asymptomatic or will substantially improve within 1 month. Therefore, it is reasonable to wait if the pain can be relieved and if the patient does not have a major neurologic deficit. The standard teaching in neurosurgery and orthopedics has been to wait 2 weeks, although I do not believe this is long enough. Many patients will improve substantially in the first month so I try to wait 1 month before proceeding with surgery for most patients. If they are improving, it is worth waiting longer because only a few patients with disk herniation fail to improve and need surgery.

There is no evidence that physical therapy or any other kind of treatment will improve the chances of avoiding surgery. This is at variance with traditional teaching, which proposes a course of physical therapy for all such patients. However, our newest data suggest that this is not beneficial. It is important to relieve pain and this may require narcotics for short periods of time. Muscle relaxants and anti-inflammatory drugs may be useful. Many neurosurgeons use a short course of corticosteroids, such as can be obtained by the Medrol Dosepak™, which is a convenient form of administration. Many patients who receive corticosteroids for a week or so will feel much better. Some clinicians use epidural corticosteroid injections around the involved root, although this can entail complications such as epidural punctures that cause nerve injury, pseudomeningocele (herniation of the arachnoid through an inadvertent puncture site through the dura), and substantial epidural scarring that can complicate subsequent surgery. Therefore, I do not routinely recommend this technique.

How long to wait before surgery depends on the patient's symptoms. If the patient is severely incapacitated, it is best to proceed with surgery immediately. But with patients who can function, I prefer to wait at least 1 month. If no improvement has occurred, then surgery should proceed. If the patient is improving, there is sufficient reason to wait longer. Surgery can always be carried out if the patient plateaus at an unacceptable level.

What Can I Do While I Am Waiting?

Patients always ask this question. Bed rest should be used only as long as the patient requires it; usually, a few days is enough to eliminate the acutely painful phase. If analgesics are effective, mobilize patients immediately and keep them active, even letting them go back to work if that does not require duties that are unusually stressful on the spine. Advise them to limit lifting, strenuous activities of all kinds, and to avoid sports or anything else that produces axial loading. Otherwise, let them return to normal activity with the admonition to quit any activity that makes their back and leg hurt.

There is no evidence that the time-honored prescriptions of prolonged bed rest, hospital lumbar traction, home traction, and prolonged restrictions of activities are beneficial. Warn patients that if an acute flare-up of pain occurs, or if neurologic deficits or any new neurologic changes occur, they should call their physician.

Techniques of Surgery on the Lumbar Spine

Surgical procedures on the lumbar spine correct only two abnormalities,[6,7] compression of nerve roots and mechanical instability. The most common reason for surgery is a disk herniation with compression of one or more nerve roots. Spinal stenosis with cauda equina syndrome is rapidly increasing because of the ease of diagnosis with MRI. Spinal fusion is indicated for demonstrated instability.

Lumbar diskectomy. Surgery on the lumbar disk is indicated when sciatic pain is intractable, when there are associated neurologic deficits of functional significance, or when there is significant weakness or loss of bowel and bladder function. The typical herniated disk begins with the acute onset of sciatica with or without back pain. Neurologic deficits may occur, but more commonly pain is the only symptom. Most patients recover spontaneously in 1 to 3 months. For most patients surgery should be delayed at least 2 weeks, preferably 4, and, if possible, 12. During this period most patients will recover spontaneously and not need further treatment. However, if spontaneous recovery does not occur, the diagnosis should be verified

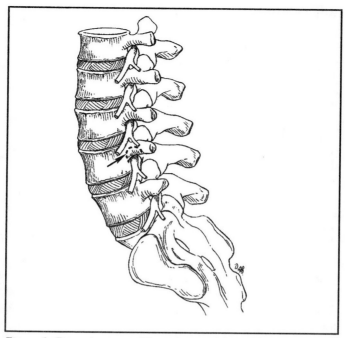

Figure 1: Foraminotomy. The arrow and dotted line depict bony removal required to open the neural foramen, accomplished from medial to lateral. This simply shows the bone that will be removed to achieve nerve-root decompression.

by MRI or CT-myelogram and surgery can proceed without physical therapy measures. While spontaneous recovery is the rule, there is no evidence that the addition of therapy improves the natural recovery.

Disk herniations may be of several types, but all compress the nerve root or cauda equina. The free fragment disk denotes rupture of a fragment of nucleus through the annulus into the epidural space. A bulging disk refers to a fragment of nucleus that has herniated from the interspace, but is still contained by an intact ligament. Diffuse disk bulges are common and do not necessarily have significance. Root compression must be demonstrated.

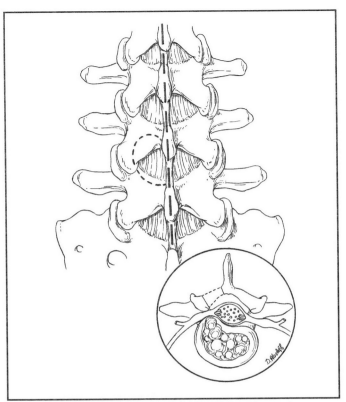

Figure 2: Hemilaminectomy. The dotted line shows the approximate amount of bone removal required for hemilaminectomy to resect a herniated disk. The insert demonstrates the disk protrusion compressing the spinal nerve in the neural foramen.

Other causes of root compression exist. The nerve root may be compromised by a spur, by thickened bulging annulus, by a stenotic foramen, by ligament, or by synovial cyst. Imaging studies are now effective in delineating all of these conditions. The clinical syndrome depends on the compressed root and does not vary with diagnosis.

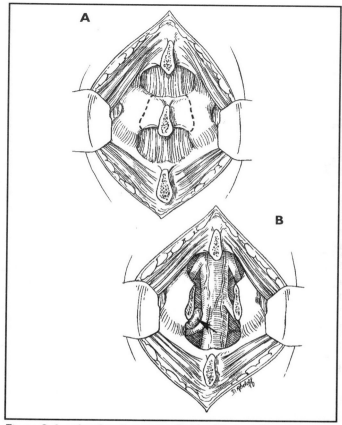

Figure 3: Lumbar Laminectomy (A,B). (A) A midline skin incision has been made. The muscles are retracted to expose the laminae. Dotted lines depict the area removed in laminectomy. (B) Composite drawing shows the bony removal of laminectomy and the typical location of a herniated disk. Laminectomy would not be required for disk removal, which would be carried out without such extensive bone removal.

Once it is certain the patient will not recover spontaneously, usually after 1 to 3 months, surgery should proceed. The opera-

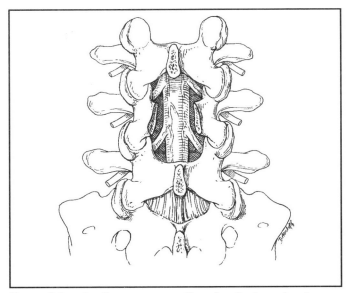

Figure 4: Lumbar Laminectomy. Drawing depicts what is required for complete laminectomy. The nerve roots are followed through their respective foramina. This procedure is called foraminotomy.

tion can be carried out under local or general anesthesia. Typically, the procedure requires 1 to several days in the hospital and about 2 weeks of relative incapacitation. Most patients return to sedentary activity after 2 weeks and full activity after 4 to 6 weeks. Heavy labor and strenuous exertion should be limited for at least 6 weeks and, although experts disagree, it is typical for patients to be kept from the most strenuous exertion for 3 to 6 months after diskectomy.

The technique requires exposure of the interspace and removal of a small amount of bone to allow access to the epidural space through the ligamentum flavum. The disk and whatever remains within the disk space is removed from the interspace. Although it is impossible to remove all the lumbar disk, as much degenerated nucleus as possible should be removed. Recovery is

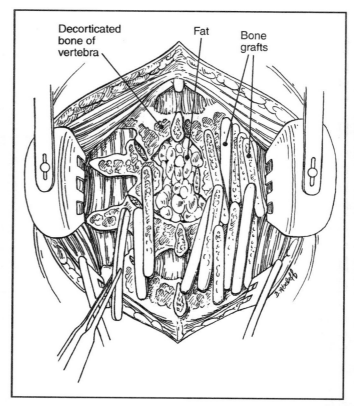

Figure 5: Lumbar Laminectomy. When fusion is required, the bone exposed is decorticated with a drill and multiple bone grafts are laid in the area to obtain posterolateral fusion.

usually prompt, and patients commonly are pain free when they awake from surgery.

Microdiskectomy. Microdiskectomy is the use of an operating microscope or magnification to carry out the operation. The magnification allows for less exposure and emphasizes gentle tissue handling. There are no data to suggest that the outcome of surgery is dramatically improved.

When the problem is other than simple disk herniation, *foraminotomy* may be required (Figure 1). This means enlarging the neural foramen to be sure there is no nerve compression from any extraneous source. Foraminotomy may also be a part of simple diskectomy when compression is caused by more than just disk herniation.

Lumbar Laminectomy (Figures 3,4,5). The disk is removed through what is generally termed hemilaminectomy (Figure 2), which means part of one lamina on one side is removed. The term laminectomy means that both laminae (right and left) and the spinous process are removed to decompress the spinal canal. The procedure is usually done for spinal stenosis and the cauda equina syndrome.

More complex than simple diskectomy, this procedure is done with general anesthesia and patients typically stay in the hospital 3 to 5 days. The goal of surgery is decompression of the spinal canal and the nerve roots in the foramina.

Outcome of Lumbar Diskectomy and Laminectomy

More than 90% of patients who undergo surgery on the herniated lumbar disk achieve immediate relief and remain asymptomatic or nearly so. Five to 10% of patients require additional surgery in the next 2 to 5 years, but most do not suffer recurrence.

Complications include sensory loss, paralysis, or severe pain from nerve injury. A rare complication is infection of the disk. The syndrome of *diskitis* is characterized by the onset of severe back pain after surgery. The white count and the sedimentation rate are elevated, and patients generally have intractable back pain. Most of these patients are seriously ill and the combination of excruciating pain with elevated white count and sedimentation rate will confirm the diagnosis. Radionuclide scans are positive. A simple bone scan will be positive after surgery so a more specific gallium or indium scan is necessary. Direct culture is successful only occasionally by the percutaneous route and even at the time of surgery culture of the organism is not always possible. Treatment is appropriate antibiotic therapy for 1 to 6 months until symptoms resolve. If a mass lesion appears, surgical drainage may be necessary. Surgery is indicated for significant neurologic deficit or intractable pain.

Rarely, the instruments used to remove the disk from the interspace can protrude into the retroperitoneal space and injure the bowel, great vessels, or ureter. Postoperative hematoma could produce a cauda equina syndrome. Cerebrospinal fluid leak is another rare complication. The complications of laminectomy are virtually the same, but surgically-induced instability is more likely to occur after the more extensive procedure.

Chemonucleolysis

In an attempt to avoid direct surgery, dissolution of the disk by injection of an enzyme that destroys the nucleus was introduced many years ago. The technique has never gained much popularity, but is still used by a few experts. The principal advantage is that it does not require a surgical incision because the enzyme can be introduced under fluoroscopic control into the nucleus percutaneously. In well-chosen patients, the success rate is only slightly less than that for surgical diskectomy. The technique is most useful in the diffusely bulging disk. The principal complication is anaphylaxis and this potentially fatal side effect has reduced the popularity of the technique.

Percutaneous Diskectomy

Another percutaneous method is percutaneous diskectomy or nucleotomy. In this technique, a large-bore needle is introduced percutaneously into the lumbar disk space to remove as much of the nucleus as possible by a guillotine-type device or by laser. Controlled trials are not yet available, but analysis suggests that the outcome of the technique is less effective than that reported for surgical diskectomy. A significant number of patients eventually require direct surgery. Patients who would be candidates for chymopapain injection are generally thought to be candidates for percutaneous diskectomy. While the technique is common, not enough comparative data exist to judge its relative merits versus standard diskectomy. It appears that some patients may avoid open surgery if percutaneous diskectomy is used, but the failure rate is high enough that many patients must undergo surgery.

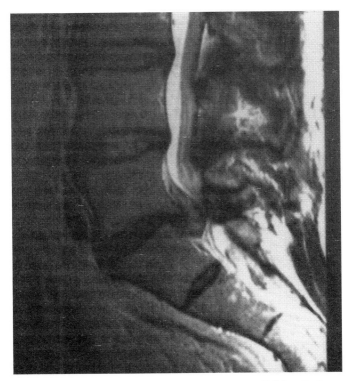

Figure 6: Lateral MRI demonstrates an enormous disk herniation at the L5-S1 space. The free-fragment disk is still contained by the ligament, but is completely out of the interspace.

Fusion of the Lumbar Spine

Lumbosacral fusion is indicated for demonstrated instability, but its use is controversial and experts disagree about its indications. Fusion is commonly employed under some specific circumstances:

(1) *Isthmic spondylolisthesis.* In this condition there is a bilateral, usually symmetrical, defect in the pars interarticularis, allowing the spine to move. The problem is equally common in men and women, virtually always occurs at L5-S1, and is easily

recognized with imaging studies (Figure 6). Symptoms include back pain with leg pain usually in the L5 distribution. Surgical fusion is nearly always indicated when the symptoms are serious. Surgical outcome is excellent.

(2) *Degenerative spondylolisthesis.* This problem occurs mostly in women at L4-5 and may also be associated with L4 or L5 root compression syndromes. There is less certainty about which patients should get this fusion technique. Progressive instability is rare, so fusion is generally reserved for those with demonstrated movement of 4 mm or more on flexion/extension films. However, some advocate the liberal policy of fusing most of these patients. There is no agreement about clear indications for fusion in this disease.

(3) *Surgical defect of the spine.* During surgery the pars interarticularis is commonly divided or the facet joint is destabilized by removal of part of the articular surface. In such circumstances cervical fusion of the involved area may be required.

(4) *Scoliosis, rotoscoliosis,* and *lateral translation* are mechanical abnormalities that indicate a slowly progressive spinal instability. Fusion is usually carried out when the abnormality is both painful and progressive.

Types of Lumbar Fusion

A number of lumbar fusions are available. The choice is usually based on the degree of instability and the anatomic abnormality being corrected. The simplest surgical technique uses local or hip graft bone to pack around the bony surfaces exposed in the course of decompressive surgery. A variation of this technique is termed posterolateral fusion and requires that the transverse processes also be exposed and the bone laid between them.

Internal Fixators for Lumbar Fusion

Several kinds of metal devices are available to stabilize the lumbar spine. These devices provide immediate stability and allow correction of anatomic abnormalities. Those available by posterior route include transarticular screws, several kinds of laminar rods, and the pedicle screw system (Figure 7) in which fixating screws are placed through the pedicle into the vertebral

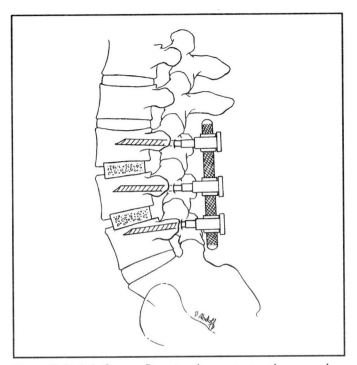

Figure 7: Pedicle Screw. Drawing demonstrates the general principles of two types of fusion. First, bony grafts have been placed in the interspace after disk removal. This may be done by the anterior or posterior approach and is termed interbody fusion. Second, the pedicle-screw system is shown with the screws placed down through the pedicles into the cortex of the vertebral body, with interlocking devices used posteriorly to stabilize the spine. These would be supplemented by bone fusion.

body, stabilizing the spine by posterior plates fastened between these screws. There is still much debate about when these techniques should be used. Their principal goal is immediate stability with an increased chance of eventual solid bony union. Their exact role in lumbar surgery is still being explored.

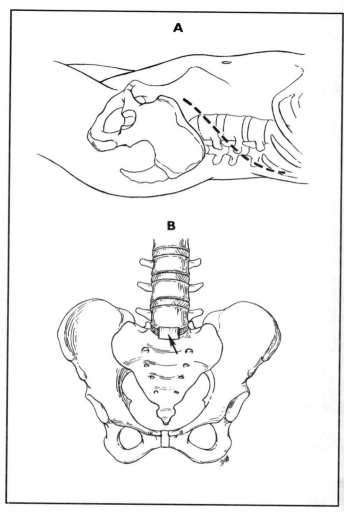

Figure 8: Anterior Approach - Lumbar Fusion (A,B). (A) Depiction of the lateral approach, which is a retroperitoneal exposure. (B) Demonstration of the place where the bone graft will be inserted in the disk space after disk removal.

Anterior Fusion Techniques for the Lumbar Spine

The lumbar spine can be fused from the front. A retroperitoneal exposure is carried out and the lumbar disks can be identified after some mobilization of distal aorta and iliac vessels with the vena cava. Disk removal is straightforward. Fusion with bone or with metal fixators has been described. The technique is generally reserved for expert spinal surgeons and is not a common practice (Figure 8).

Complications of Lumbar Fusion

Fusion is a more complicated operation than straightforward diskectomy or laminectomy. Failure occurs in 5% to 15% of fusion patients. The infection rate and risk of nerve injury are somewhat higher and the complications of misplaced hardware are significant. Patients require longer hospital stays and longer time to recover. A typical patient does not begin recovery until 3 months and is not fully recovered until 6 months. Outcome of fusion in terms of pain relief is generally good.

Facet Arthropathy and the So-called Facet Denervation

Spondylitic arthritic change in the facet joints can be painful. The facet arthropathy is easily imaged. Patients typically have back pain without a sciatic component. The diagnosis is made by anesthetization of the involved joints. When pain relief is induced by these facet blocks, the diagnosis is probable. A variety of techniques has been used to try to permanently denervate the painful joints. They are innervated by the medial branch of the posterior primary ramus of the exiting spinal nerve and the one immediately above. The most common technique is radiofrequency destruction of these nerves where they cross the root of the transverse process. This is typically called facet denervation or facet rhizolysis. Some spinal experts use the technique, but rarely. There are no controlled series of patients in the literature, but case reports suggest that the technique is effective in well-chosen patients. It plays a limited role in the overall management of low back pain, however. Only a small number of patients appear to have pain that is generated principally from the zygapophyseal joints.

Table 1: Causes of Failed Back Syndrome

- Lack of appropriate indications for surgery initially
- Cause of pain not identified appropriately before the first procedure
- Postoperative scarring

Failed back syndrome is a nonspecific term that connotes more than two lumbar surgeries without pain relief. The causes are many. Imaging studies are the key to diagnosis, but history of the pain can be helpful. A radicular pattern of pain suggests nerve root compression or injury. Nonradicular leg pain may occur without ongoing root compression. This is generally termed referred pain, but no one is certain of the etiology. Back pain only suggests instability. Virtually all patients are worsened by activity and improved by rest and nearly all are significantly limited in their physical activities.

The first imaging study should be lumbosacral spine films with flexion and extension. It is important to understand the extent of the previous surgical defect, particularly looking for evidence of spondylolisthesis, defects in the zygapophyseal joints, or defects in the pars interarticularis. If previous fusion has been attempted, the quality of the fusion should be assessed. MRI, which has replaced virtually all other studies for the patient who has not had surgery, is less definitive in the patient who has had multiple previous operations. Still, it appears to be the single best test if no hardware is present. If bony abnormalities are suspected or found on plain films, then CT scan with two- and three-dimensional reconstructions will define them accurately. Both also reduce metal artifact in the images. Electromyography (EMG), which has virtually no role in diagnosis of the acutely herniated disk, may be helpful in these patients. It may be possible to identify an injured root as well as signs of root recovery. Because these patients often have bilateral symptoms, differentiating polyneuropathy can be important. The EMG is still used selectively and for a minority of patients, but it has greater impact here than elsewhere in lumbar spine diagnosis.

Causes of failed back syndrome are listed in Table 1. The most common cause is lack of appropriate indications for surgery initially. When the patient was not a good candidate for the first surgery, it is not surprising that subsequent operations are not beneficial. The cause of the pain was not identified appropriately before the first procedure, which did not address the patient's problem.

Postoperative scarring is probably the most common physical cause and is generally not amenable to surgical repair. Reoperation can benefit nerve compression or spinal instability. When the evaluation demonstrates compression of nerve root by recurrent disk, a mass-like scar, bony spurring, or foraminal compression, then surgery is likely to be beneficial. When instability is found, fusion will successfully relieve pain. Some surgeons tend to offer fusion when an initial surgery fails in the absence of clearly demonstrated instability. Such a procedure is unlikely to help the patient.

The outcome of reoperative surgery depends entirely on the condition to be corrected. Second operations are generally as effective as first-time procedures. The success rate of third operations and beyond is less. In our extensive experience, satisfactory outcome is achieved about 60% of the time, but many patients retain residual disability.

When reoperation is not indicated or fails, spinal cord stimulation remains a possible treatment.

Rehabilitation of the Patient With Failed Back Syndrome

Evidence indicates that many patients suffering from residual pain after multiple operations can benefit from an intensive rehabilitation program. Conventional manipulation and passive therapy measures are of no value. However, an intensive rehabilitation program that focuses on stretching and eliminating local inflammatory changes, spinal muscle strengthening, general reconditioning, and improvement of function will be successful. Most patients will have improved functioning with less pain. However, in my experience complete elimination of pain and disability by any of these techniques is not a realistic goal and patients must be aware of the aims of therapy, whether rehabilitation or surgery, so that they do not have unrealistic expectations.

References

1. Cailliet R: *Low Back Pain Syndrome*. 4th ed. Philadelphia, FA Davis Co, 1988.

2. Nachemson AL: The lumbar spine: an orthopedic challenge. *Spine* 1976;1:59.

3. Burton CV, et al: Causes of failure of surgery on the lumbar spine. *Clin Orthop* 1981;157:191-199.

4. Waddell G: A new clinical model for the treatment of low back pain. *Spine* 1987;12:632-644.

5. Lewis PJ, et al: Long-term prospective study of lumbosacral diskectomy. *J Neurosurg* 1987;67:49-53.

6. Weber H: Lumbar disk herniation. A controlled prospective study with ten years of observation. *Spine* 1983;8:131-140.

7. Spangfort EV: The lumbar disk herniation. A computer-aided analysis of 2,504 operations. *Acta Orthop Scand* 1972(suppl);142:1-95.

Chapter 6

Neuropathic Pain

Clinical Characteristics of Neuropathic Pain

Pain associated with injury to the nervous system is called neuropathic pain.[1] The most common causes are injury to peripheral nerves, spinal cord injury, and stroke. A number of other specific problems will be described in this chapter. Despite the diverse origins of neuropathic pain, all of these syndromes share certain characteristics that are typical enough to diagnose neuropathic pain when they are reported by the patient. These features allow neuropathic pain to be separated from tissue-destructive processes in which nervous system function is normal.

Patients characteristically describe neuropathic pain as burning, lancinating, constant, unrelieved by rest, associated with paresthesias and, even more typically, dysesthesias. Patients find these sensations extremely disturbing. Increased sensory input or change in sensation, such as application of heat or cold, often cause the pain to worsen, as does emotional upset. Narcotics are not generally effective treatments.

On physical examination, the hallmarks of neuropathic pain are neurologic abnormalities.[2] Typically, there is both loss of sensation and disordered sensation. Paradoxically, a patient may have hypesthesia to one modality and hyperesthesia to another. Light touch and change in temperature characteristically worsen the pain. The hyperesthesia may be so severe that patients cannot even tolerate bedclothes on an affected limb. There is often weakness that may be secondary to direct injury or to trophic changes, which is another hallmark of the disease. Muscle atrophy is often out of proportion to apparent motor injury. Trophic changes in the skin, including lack of sweating or excessive sweating and a thin, shiny skin, are common. Autonomic changes are also common. The involved area of denervation is often hot or cold, sometimes paradoxically so. Local blood flow is often affected.

Pathophysiology of Neuropathic Pain

Much debate exists about the changes that underline neuropathic pain. Clinicians generally agree that sensations may be short-circuited from one fiber to another in the area of injury, which is called ephaptic transmission. Ectopic impulses may begin spontaneously in the area of injury rather than in a specific receptor more peripherally. Activation of the innervation of the nerve itself (nervi-nervorum) is another suspected mechanism. Denervation hypersensitivity may occur, whereby denervated or partially denervated receptors become especially sensitive to circulating transmitters. It has also been suggested that the injury causes disinhibition of central pain transmission neurons, which are commonly kept in balance by the painful and nonpainful signals coming in. This imbalance can lead to excessive activity in the pain system.[3]

A classic neuropathic pain is so-called *reflex sympathetic dystrophy*.[4] This term, which is still common in the literature, is no longer used. Instead, *sympathetically mediated pain* is now used. This peculiar syndrome was originally described in Civil War veterans who had suffered gunshot wounds of major peripheral nerves. The term in use for many years was "causalgia." Researchers in the early part of this century recognized that dysesthetic pain after peripheral nerve injury could often be temporarily relieved by sympathetic blockade and cured by surgical sympathectomy. This became standard treatment. But sympathectomy was not always effective. We now know that this is simply another form of neuropathic pain in which reflex activation of the pain system occurs through the sympathetic nervous system. Interruption of the sympathetic nervous system breaks the reflex arch, and so relieves the pain. Chemical percutaneous blockade has been the standard method of diagnosing the syndrome for many years. Now there are alternatives. Intravenous infusion of phentolamine (Regitine®) mimics chemical sympathetic blockade and produces the same pain relief in sympathetically mediated pain. Surgical sympathectomy is still the best treatment, but an equivalent effect can sometimes be obtained by medication. Mexiletine (Mexitil®) 150 mg b.i.d. taken with food up to 10 mg/kg/day administered orally will frequently provide lasting relief for these patients.

Common Neuropathic Pain Syndromes

Painful Mononeuropathies. The most common of these are the nerve root compression syndromes from disk herniation or spondylotic disease (described in Chapter 5). Similar symptoms can occur from involvement of a major plexus. Neoplastic infiltration of the lumbosacral plexus or the brachial plexus results in a neuropathic syndrome involving the upper or lower extremity.[5]

Of course, individual nerves may be affected. The most typical are median compression at the wrist (carpal tunnel syndrome) and compression of the ulnar nerve at the elbow (tardy ulnar palsy). Other entrapment neuropathies affect individual nerves, and most require an expert in peripheral nerve disease for diagnosis. However, carpal tunnel syndrome and tardy ulnar palsy are common and straightforward to diagnose. Carpal tunnel syndrome is characterized by neuropathic pain involving the thumb and lateral two fingers of the affected hand. Sensory loss occurs in the distribution of the median nerve, usually in the thumb, and the same two fingers. Thumb weakness and atrophy of the thenar eminence is obvious. The pain is frequently dysesthetic. Diagnosis is made by history and by electromyographic evidence of compression of the nerve at the wrist.

Tardy ulnar palsy is characterized by pain involving the lateral half of the fourth and fifth fingers. The pain is commonly dysesthetic and is associated with atrophy in the hypothenar eminence and intrinsic muscles of the hand. Compression of the ulnar nerve at the elbow often reproduces symptoms. Nerve conduction studies are diagnostic.

The treatment for mild symptoms in both conditions is splinting in a functional position. When the symptoms are more severe or not relieved by splinting, surgical decompression is usually curative.

Painful Polyneuropathy. Most polyneuropathies can be painful. Diabetes and alcoholism are commonly associated with severe neuropathic pain. In general, the pain is in a stocking-glove distribution, although mononeuropathies do occur. Trophic changes and burning dysesthesias are typical. Increasing sensory input usually worsens the pain, which is particularly disabling at night. These conditions must be differentiated from cervical and/or spinal canal stenosis.[5]

The Neuroma. Peripheral nerve injury naturally leads to neuroma formation.[2] Many neuromas are not painful, but some are exquisitely sensitive and generate severe pain with any mechanical distortion. Even moving or touching the area of a nerve injury may be very painful. The neuroma usually can be palpated and lightly tapping it brings on the pain. Typically, neuromas occur in amputation stumps, but they may develop in nerves in an intact extremity. The diagnosis is suspected by the history and the tenderness of the area of injury. Usually, the neuroma can be palpated, but sometimes it requires surgical exploration. The typical syndrome is amputation stump pain. This must be differentiated from phantom pain, which is not local to the stump but in the imaginary amputated extremity. Other surgical syndromes are also probably caused by neuromas. Postmastectomy pain is generally secondary to nerve root entrapment or neuromas generated from the radical surgery. Postthoracotomy syndrome, which is pain in the distribution of the thoracotomy incision, also results from nerve injury. Treatment has been surgical excision so that the new neuroma that forms is less exposed and not so easily traumatized.

Deafferentation Pain Syndromes. So-called central pain is often called deafferentation pain. It arises from injuries in the nervous system or from changes that occur within the nervous system that are related to more peripheral injuries. Five categories of deafferentation pain are common enough to require description.

Phantom pain. Many patients who undergo amputation, particularly after traumatic injury to an extremity, develop a painful distortion of the phantom limb.[6] Virtually all patients who lose extremities have the ongoing sensation that the limb is still present. For most, this sensation is not painful, but for some, it is continuously painful. While the exact mechanisms have yet to be defined, it is generally accepted that changes in receptive fields within the central nervous system account for this phenomenon. Treatment is by medications, described later in this chapter, that have a reasonable chance of relieving the pain. Some patients have also been treated by deep brain stimulation.

Postherpetic neuralgia. Postherpetic neuralgia is another central pain phenomenon. Typically, patients have had a bout of herpes zoster that is acutely painful. A few patients develop neuropathic pain in the area of the previous eruption. There is usually marked dysesthesia of the skin and constant pain. The pain is often worsened by lancinating episodes of severe, tic-like pain. Postherpetic neuralgia has been notoriously difficult to treat. Recent data suggest that unlike most neuropathic pains, it can be managed well with long-term narcotics. Alternatives include the general drugs used for neuropathic pain.[7]

Brachial plexus avulsion. Pain that occurs with avulsion of the brachial plexus is typical,[8] obvious from the history of trauma with the development of a flail upper extremity. Most patients have a functionless arm although small amounts of residual nerve function can occasionally be present. The diagnosis is made with electrical studies and when the MRI shows the dural pouches that typically occur with the avulsion injury. The pain is like phantom pain except that the limb is still present. The patient often perceives the limb to be distorted and the dysesthetic sensations are particularly disagreeable. The pain is often worsened by any manipulation of the limb even though it is apparently completely denervated. Brachial plexus avulsion pain was virtually untreatable for many years, but the development of surgical destruction of the involved dorsal root entry zone area has revolutionized treatment. The operation is nearly always successful and the risks of accompanying neurologic deficits are small. This severe pain is now among the easiest of all pain problems to treat.

Pain of spinal cord injury origin. Most patients who have significant spinal cord injury complain of dysesthesias and paresthesias felt below the level of the injury. Only a few have dysesthesias so unpleasant as to be termed "pain." The diagnosis is usually obvious. The dysesthesias are widespread in all the denervated area below the level of injury. The pain is not local. This is important because an unstable, poorly healed fracture is a common cause of local pain in a spinal injury. Rather, these patients have diffuse burning pain throughout the body below the level of injury. A small number of patients achieve pain relief from spinal cord stimulation, but most are best treated by medications.[9]

Thalamic pain. Some patients who have strokes that principally involve sensory portions of thalamus and/or internal capsule develop neuropathic pain on the side opposite the stroke. Characteristically, such patients have a motor sensory stroke with both loss of sensation and paralysis. However, the sensory loss predominates and paralysis frequently improves dramatically. Patients are left with profound sensory loss and painful dysesthesias involving all of the parts of the body affected by the stroke, including the face alone or any body part on the entire side of the body opposite the stroke. The pain is characteristically described as "burning" and may be worsened by sensory input or emotional upset. The treatment is usually medical. Some patients are treated with deep brain stimulation, but the injury from the stroke often precludes the use of any central procedure.[10]

Sympathetically Mediated Pain Syndromes (Reflex Sympathetic Dystrophy)

The key to making the diagnosis is usually the history of peripheral nerve or substantial peripheral soft-tissue injury.[11] The diagnosis is suspected from the history and from the neuropathic character of the pain. There is nothing specific about the pain. It has the common features of neuropathic pain. Plain x-rays may show demineralization of bone; a radioactive bone scan may be positive in the abnormal areas. The best diagnostic test is sympathetic blockade, which can be done by direct injection of the sympathetic trunk or by intravenous phentolamine. The diagnosis of sympathetically mediated pain is made when pain is relieved. However, remember that because single blocks may be misleading, repeated blocks are needed to confirm the diagnosis. Surgical sympathectomy is effective treatment, but medical sympathectomy can also be employed.

Medical Therapy for Neuropathic Pain

Fortunately, several categories of drugs may be successful in treating any of the forms of neuropathic pain (Tables 1-6). In general, these pains do not respond to narcotics and that may be one of the important diagnostic points. Most drugs used for neuropathic pain have only anecdotal evidence about efficacy. A few clinical trials have been done in postherpetic neuralgia and diabetic neuropathy, but the use of the other drugs rests principally on anecdotal evidence reported by experts in the field.

The drugs in most common use are amitriptyline (Elavil®), carbamazepine (Tegretol®), and clonazepam (Klonopin®). These drugs require trials of several weeks. I usually begin with one and escalate the dose until there is successful alleviation of pain, failure to relieve the pain, or the development of substantial side effects. Typically, after 3 weeks of trying a drug without success, that drug should be discontinued and a second begun.

Amitriptyline. The use of this drug for pain control is probably the best established of any of the techniques. Controlled trials have demonstrated its usefulness in postherpetic neuralgia and diabetic neuropathy. Begin with 25 mg to 50 mg at bedtime. This allows the sedative effect to aid the impaired sleeping that so commonly accompanies neuropathic pain syndrome. If no relief has occurred after 1 week, double the dose to 100 mg to 150 mg at bedtime. Side effects include blurred vision, dry mouth, constipation, urinary retention, and somnolence. If side effects occur, the drug must be discontinued. If effective, the dose is simply titrated to the lowest dose that provides lasting relief.

Carbamazepine. This drug is used routinely for neuropathic pain. Phenytoin (Dilantin®) is also used, but carbamazepine is more effective. The initial dose should be 200 mg per day for 2 to 3 days and then the dose is increased in 200-mg increments over 1 week to a total of 600 mg to 800 mg per day. There is no

Table 1: Systemic Medications for Neuropathic Pain

• **Nonsteroidal anti-inflammatory drugs (NSAIDs):** Aleve®, Anaprox®, Cataflam®, IBU®, Lodine®, Motrin®, Nalfon®, Naprosyn®, Ponstel®, Relafen®, Toradol®

• **Opiates:** Anexsia®, DHCplus®, Darvocet-N®, Darvon®, Demerol®, Dilaudid®, Empirin® with Codeine, Fioricet® with Codeine, Fiorinal® with Codeine, Hydrocet®, Levo-Dromoran®, Lorcet®, Lortab®, MS Contin®, MSIR®, Methadone, Oramorph SR™, Percocet®, Percodan®, Roxanol™, Roxicet™, Roxicodone™, Talwin® Nx, Tylenol® with Codeine, Tylox®, Vicodin®, Wygesic®, Zydone®, OxyContin™

• **Antidepressants:** Asendin®, Elavil®, Endep®, Etrafon®, Limbitrol®, Norpramin®, Pamelor®, Sinequan®, Surmontil®, Tofranil®, Triavil®, Vivactil®

• **Tramadol:** Ultram®

• **Anticonvulsants:** Atretol®, Celontin®, Depakene®, Depakote®, Diamox®, Dilantin®, Felbatol®, Klonopin®, Lamictal®, Mebaral®, Mesantoin®, Milontin®, Mysoline®, Nembutal®, Neurontin®, Peganone®, Phenobarbital, Phenurone®, Tegretol®, Tranxene®, Valium®, Zarontin®

• **Antiarrhythmic agents:** Adenocard®, Betapace®, Brevibloc®, Calan®, Cardizem®, Cordarone®, Ethmozine®, Inderal®, Isoptin®, Lanoxin®, Mexitil®, Norpace®, Procan® SR, Quinaglute Dura-Tabs®, Quinidex Extentabs®, Rythmol®, Sectral®, Tambocor®, Tonocard®

evidence that further increases are likely to be useful, but pushing the dose to side effects and then reducing the amount of drug given will certainly give the patient a thorough trial. Common side effects are excessive somnolence, change in mental status, and dry eye. The requirement to monitor the hematologic picture is no longer mandatory, but an occasional patient will develop

Table 2: Systemic Medications: Anticonvulsants

Mechanisms: Membrane stabilization
Sodium channel inhibition

- Carbamazepine (Atretol®, Tegretol®)
- Gabapentin (Neurontin®)
- Clonazepam (Klonopin®)
- Valproate (Depakene®) and phenytoin (Dilantin®)

Table 3: Systemic Medications: Antiarrhythmic Agents

- Lidocaine (Decadron®, Xylocaine®): Infusions up to 5 mg/kg may give long-lasting effects
- Mexiletine (Mexitil®): P.O. dosing up to 10 mg/kg; Check EKG
- Bretylium: Used in Bier blocks for distal pain

profound changes in peripheral blood and so an occasional check is still worthwhile. Phenytoin is used when carbamazepine is not tolerated. I begin with 100 mg per day and escalate to 300 mg per day or to a level that would be therapeutic for seizures.

Clonazepam. For this drug, begin with 0.5 mg once a day and then escalate the dose to a total of 1.5 mg per day. The drug has few side effects, but an occasional patient will suffer mild withdrawal symptoms each morning. These may preclude the use of the drug.

Other drugs have been used, such as other antidepressants, and most find that they work. Valproate (Depakene®) is another anticonvulsant medication that seems to be effective in some patients who do not tolerate phenytoin or carbamazepine.

Table 4: Chronic Pain Treatment

Aching Pain

• Nonsteroidal anti-inflammatory drugs (Aleve®, Anaprox®, Cataflam®, IBU®, Lodine®, Motrin®, Nalfon®, Naprosyn®, Ponstel®, Relafen®, Toradol®) up to 2400 mg/day

• Tramadol (Ultram®)
    25 mg b.i.d., q.i.d. to 100 mg q.i.d.

• Opiates
Morphine (MS Contin®, MSIR®, Oramorph SR™, Roxanol™) or oxycodone (Percocet®, Percodan®, Roxicodone™, Tylox®) 5 mg q.i.d. to pain relief, or transdermal fentanyl (Duragesic®). After 30 mg per day switch to CR preparations (MS Contin® or OxyContin®), methadone, or transdermal fentanyl (Duragesic®).

Table 5: Neuropathic Pain Treatment

Burning Pain

• Tricyclic antidepressants (Asendin®, Elavil®, Endep®, Etrafon®, Limbitrol®, Norpramin®, Pamelor®, Sinequan®, Surmontil®, Tofranil®, Triavil®, Vivactil®): 10-25 mg q.h.s. to 150 mg q.d.

• Tramadol (Ultram®): 25 mg b.i.d., q.i.d. to 100 mg q.i.d.

• Gabapentin (Neurontin®): 100 mg t.i.d. to 2700 mg/day

• Mexiletine (Mexitil®): 150 mg b.i.d. to 10 mg/kg/day

• Clonazepam (Klonopin®): 0.5 mg q.h.s. to 2-3 mg/day

Sympathetically maintained pain has been treated with high doses of corticosteroids, phenoxybenzamine (Dibenzyline®), prazosin (Minipress®), and nifedipine (Adalat®, Procardia®). More recently, mexiletine has been used. In general, these drugs are still in clinical investigation and their use is best left to experts in the pain field.

Table 6: Neuropathic Pain Treatment

Lancinating Pain

• Gabapentin (Neurontin®): 100 mg t.i.d. to 2700 mg/day

• Carbamazepine (Atretol®, Tegretol®): 100 mg b.i.d. to 800 mg/day

• Tricyclic antidepressants (Asendin®, Elavil®, Endep®, Etrafon®, Limbitrol®, Norpramin®, Pamelor®, Sinequan®, Surmontil®, Tofranil®, Triavil®, Vivactil®): 10-25 mg q.h.s. to 150 mg/day

• Clonazepam (Klonopin®): 0.5 mg q.h.s. to 2-3 mg/day

• Paroxetine (Paxil®): 20 mg q.d. to 50-80 mg/day

• Mexiletine (Mexitil®): 150 mg b.i.d. to 10 mg/kg/day

Tables 1 through 6 courtesy of Donald C. Manning, MD, University of Virginia.

Surgical Procedures for Neuropathic Pain

Surgery on peripheral nerves is generally successful. Decompression of the nerve or nerve root, resection of neuromas, and the various forms of gangliolysis in trigeminal neuralgia are all effective.

Destructive procedures on the central nervous system, which are so effective in soft-tissue injury pain, are not useful in deafferentation pain syndromes. In fact, they are generally contraindicated. The exception is the dorsal root entry zone lesion, which is virtually always curative for pain of avulsion of the brachial plexus and can also be used in postherpetic neuralgia and the pain of spinal cord injury.

Spinal cord stimulation is particularly effective for neuropathic pain from injury to nerve roots or peripheral nerves. Direct nerve stimulation is an adjunctive technique used for painful mononeuropathies. Deep brain stimulation has been used for thalamic syndrome and for the pain of brain stem stroke, but the data are equivocal and the technique is no longer available.

References

1. Fields HL: Painful dysfunction of the nervous system. In: Fields HL: *Pain*. New York, McGraw-Hill Book Co, 1987, pp 133-169.

2. Sunderland S: The painful sequelae of injuries to peripheral nerves. In: Sunderland S: *Nerves and Injuries*. 2nd ed. Edinburgh, Churchill Livingstone, 1978, pp 377-420.

3. Devor M: The pathophysiology of damaged peripheral nerve. In: Wall PD, Melzack R, eds. *Textbook of Pain*. 2nd ed. Edinburgh, Churchill Livingstone, 1989, pp 63-81.

4. Payne R: Neuropathic pain syndromes, with special reference to causalgia and reflex sympathetic dystrophy. *Clin J Pain* 1986;2:59-73.

5. Scadding JW: Peripheral neuropathies. In: Wall PD, Melzack R, eds. *Textbook of Pain*. 2nd ed. Edinburgh, Churchill Livingstone, 1989, pp 522-534.

6. Sunderland S: Stump pain and abnormal sensory phenomena superimposed on the phantom state. In: Sunderland S: *Nerves and Injuries*. 2nd ed. Edinburgh, Churchill Livingstone, 1978, pp 433-447.

7. Portenoy RK, Duma C, Foley KM: Herpetic and postherpetic neuralgia: clinical review and current management. *Ann Neurol* 1986;20:651-664.

8. Wynn Parry CB: Pain in avulsion lesions of the brachial plexus. *Pain* 1980;9:40-53.

9. Pagni CA: Central pain due to spinal cord and brain stem damage. In: Wall PD, Melzack R, eds. *Textbook of Pain*. 2nd ed. Edinburgh, Churchill Livingstone, 1989, pp 634-655.

10. Tasker RR, Dostrovsky JO: Deafferentation and central pain. In: Wall PD, Melzack R, eds. *Textbook of Pain*. 2nd ed. Edinburgh, Churchill Livingstone, 1989, pp 154-180.

11. Schwartzman RJ, McLellan TL: Reflex sympathetic dystrophy, a review. *Arch Neurol* 1987;44:555-561.

////// Chapter 7

Management of Orofacial Pain

G iven the disproportionately large representation of the orofacial region in the somatosensory system, it is somewhat surprising that orofacial pain syndromes are not more common than they are. In fact, there are a relatively small number of them.

Sensation of the head is generally provided by the trigeminal nerve, although both the ninth and tenth nerves have sensory components. The upper cervical roots innervate the posterior scalp, the junction of the head and neck, and the upper neck. An abundant cervical sympathetic distribution accompanies all of the major vessels that supply the head, neck, and brain. Whatever the origin of the sensation, and regardless of which nerve the pain originates from, all pain-carrying fibers eventually enter the descending root of the trigeminal nerve. These interactions in the brain stem undoubtedly account for some of the confusing referrals of orofacial pain, such as pain felt in the face or tongue in patients with cervical disc disease.[1]

Causes of Orofacial Pain

The most common cause of orofacial pain, other than the various headache syndromes, is dental disease. Fortunately, dental pain is usually local and can be identified by examination. The temporomandibular joint syndrome and chronic sinus disease are other common causes of orofacial pain. The dura is richly innervated with pain fibers, as are the carotid arteries and the periosteum of the facial bones. While many of the syndromes involving these various structures are quite diffuse, several specific orofacial pain syndromes can be described.[2]

Dental disease. The pain is usually local around the affected tooth or at the site of abnormality. It may spread diffusely in the face, but its local origin is generally apparent and generally can be found by careful dental examination, including x-rays. Acute dental pain can be managed with nonsteroidal anti-inflammatory drugs (NSAIDs), usually aspirin or acetaminophen (Tylenol®). If stronger analgesia is required, codeine or oxycodone (Roxicodone™) are used. For severe disease, parenteral narcotics such as morphine or meperidine (Demerol®) may be required. Chronic dental pain is usually neuropathic (see Chapter 6).

Sinus disease. Most chronic sinus disease is associated with local pain and tenderness over the involved sinus. Typically, patients have a feeling of fullness or pressure, and many have postnasal drip. Examination by magnetic resonance imaging (MRI) and otolaryngology evaluation are usually diagnostic. Analgesic medication sufficient to control the pain should be used until treatment is successful.

Trigeminal neuralgia. The syndrome is typical. Trigger points bring on lancinating pain in the distribution of one or more of the branches of the trigeminal nerve. Pain can be immediately relieved by local blockade of the involved nerve. Its lancinating nature and the typical trigger points generally make the diagnosis. The pain may be in the distribution of any branch of the trigeminal nerve, but is most common in third division followed by second and first. Combinations of second and third division are common (see Chapter 11).[3]

Glossopharyngeal neuralgia. This syndrome is specific and is associated with lancinating pain in the back of the throat. The trigger is in the nasopharynx in the distribution of the ninth nerve, usually on a tonsillar pillar or in the pharynx. Occasionally, the same lancinating pain may be felt in the ear. This is a dangerous condition because the pain is sometimes associated with a dramatic decline in heart rate, even to the point of cardiac arrest. Patients often faint from the cardiac irregularity during a painful episode.

The diagnosis of glossopharyngeal neuralgia is secured by cocainization of the trigger point, which will make the pain disappear. If no significant cardiac events are present, then treatment with the same medications as used for trigeminal neuralgia, that is, carbamazepine (Tegretol®) or phenytoin (Dilantin®), will be adequate to control most patients (see Chapter 8). If there are significant cardiac events, then it is probably better to proceed to surgical therapy. Microvascular decompression has been employed. If no obviously compressive vessel is present, then cutting the nerve will solve the problem, although some patients will be left with a permanently paralyzed vocal cord and permanent hoarseness. Thus, laryngeal reparative surgery may be required and is generally very successful.

Postherpetic neuralgia. Herpes zoster characteristically involves the first division of the trigeminal nerve or the distribution of the C2 root. Other branches of the trigeminal may be involved. The problem is usually diagnosed easily because of the development of typical skin vesicles followed by pain. Rarely, postherpetic neuralgia will occur without antecedent eruption of vesicles. The pain is constant, burning, and dysesthetic. The cornea may be injured by the infection. Treatment has generally been ineffective until recently. Some clinicians believe that the persistent pain that complicates acute herpes eruptions in a small number of patients can be prevented by repeated sympathetic blocks during the acute phase. This therapy is difficult to confirm because most acute herpes infections do not result in postherpetic neuralgia.

Typically, patients develop the burning, dysesthetic pain weeks to months after the acute herpes infection is gone. The pain is severe and unrelenting, prevents sleep, and has been resistant to almost every form of therapy. However, recent good data suggest that the use of long-acting narcotics will give most of these patients satisfactory relief with minimum side effects. Long-acting narcotics, such as methadone or morphine (MS Contin®, Oramorph SR™, Roxanol™) or transdermal fentanyl (Duragesic®), are the best drugs for relief of constant and severe pain. Milder or intermittent pain is managed with NSAIDs or lesser narcotics.

The temporomandibular joint syndrome is a problem whose diagnosis and therapy are much debated. While the reality of the syndrome is not debated, its frequency is. You can easily test the validity of the syndrome by having the patient simply bite eccentrically on a pencil for 5 minutes to determine how severe the pain can be in the region of the temporomandibular joint. The problem is that some practitioners diagnose this syndrome in virtually everyone. The causes are not well understood, but appear usually to be dental. An asymmetrical bite is probably the most common cause. Typical treatment is to fit the patient with a prosthesis to correct the bite. Occasionally, true disease of the temporomandibular joint is found, but this is rare. Some have advocated the use of relaxation therapy techniques such as biofeedback to prevent patients from repetitively biting or grinding their teeth, thus reducing the stresses in the muscles of mastication. Most patients are treated effectively by dental prostheses or reparative oral surgery. NSAIDs can provide some relief, but correcting the bite is the key to control of pain.[4]

Local pain associated with *tumors of the skull base* or *vascular lesions* is rare. In general, the pain is unremitting and localized to the region of the tumor or vascular malformation. Neurological findings may or may not be present. It is unusual to confuse the pain from a specific lesion with any of the more diffuse syndromes. A good rule to follow is that when the pain is focal, an imaging study is reasonable to do. Low-grade malignancy at the base of the skull is commonly associated with persistent local pain, but other kinds of tumors, such as meningiomas, are not. If the patient has local pain that persists and does not seem to fit any of the more typical syndromes, then an imaging study should be done to investigate the cause.

A bigger problem occurs in patients with typical syndromes when a tumor is subsequently discovered. Commonly, these are meningiomas. It is unlikely that the meningiomas have anything to do with the more diffuse syndromes; instead, they are more likely to be accidental associations. The possibility is remote that the tumor is triggering migraine or some other specific syndrome. It is not worthwhile to conduct imaging studies for every patient unless something atypical suggests an intracranial or skull-base lesion.

Atypical Facial Pain

Atypical facial pain covers all of the other orofacial pain that does not fit a more specific syndrome. Patients with atypical facial pain have exactly that. They usually complain of pain that does not fit any anatomical distribution. It is frequently diffuse, distressing, and burning. Teeth are often painful. Patients may complain that the face feels numb. Neurologic deficits are not common, but when they occur they suggest a structural lesion. When a neurologic deficit is present, an imaging study should be done. But for most patients with atypical facial pain, no cause is ever found. There is a general presumption that atypical facial pain is neuropathic pain, and treated as such (see Chapter 6). There are no known surgical therapies. The treatment is medical.

Examination of the Patient With Facial Pain

The first step is to examine the patient's nervous system because structural lesions are the most important diagnoses to exclude. The examination should include all the cranial nerves, sensation of the head and neck, and visible oropharynx. Specific tests for the teeth include tooth percussion, assessment of vitality, and diagnostic blocks. The temporalis and masseter muscles can be palpated, as can the upper cervical musculature. Plain x-rays will demonstrate bony abnormality. MRI scans are highly sensitive for the sinuses and can be used to assess the rest of the tissues of the head and neck. Occasionally, specific diagnostic blocks are required, but most of the diagnoses are either straightforward and do not require additional diagnostic studies or are nonspecific. Nerve blocks are not beneficial in improving specificity.

Headache

Headache is the most common of all pain syndromes, occurring more frequently than low back pain. Most headaches are nondescript and require symptomatic treatment, but a few are specific, and require specific therapies. Because headache is so common, all physicians must understand appropriate diagnosis and management.[5]

Anatomic and Physiologic Features Relevant to Headache

Headache may arise from cervical musculature or disk disease, instability of upper cervical facet joints, structural abnormalities, diseases of the skull, sinus disease, dural injury, and increased intracranial pressure. Some headaches apparently arise in the vascular system, and many have no discernible anatomic abnormalities. The pain may come from the vascular system supplying the head and neck, from the dura and pericranium, from the teeth and temporomandibular joints, and from sinuses. Destructive lesions anywhere at the base of the skull cause head pain.[5]

The trigeminal sensory system is responsible for innervation of most of the head and neck. The ninth and tenth cranial nerves play a role in the oropharynx and posterior fossa dura. The upper cervical cranial nerves supply the back of the head, lateral side of the head, and part of the ear, as well as upper cervical joints.

The cephalic vascular system is richly innervated from both sympathetics and parasympathetics. Vessels in dura have demonstrated pain fibers. It is less certain that those in the brain have these pain-carrying fibers. The cerebral vasculature has a rich sympathetic system that arises in all three cervical ganglia, and then follows both internal and external carotid systems, as well as the vertebrals.

Hypotheses concerning the mechanisms of headaches can be divided into three general categories: (1) myofascial or skeletal mechanisms from the cervical spine; (2) abnormalities of blood flow to the brain; and (3) a variety of diseases involving the face, including the temporomandibular joint syndrome and chronic sinusitis.

Historical Examination for Headache

Much can be learned from the patient's history. The physical examination is generally unrewarding, but the history will often make the diagnosis. It is important to know the frequency and the duration of the attacks, as well as anything the patient has identified that may precipitate the headache. Constant, unremitting pain suggests intracranial pressure. Pain related to physical activity, particularly when it originates in the neck, is often cervical in origin. The relationship of headaches to foodstuffs suggests migraine, as does hemicranial headache. Cervical headaches are generally suboccipital and involve the C2 and C3 distribution. Headache associated with increased intracranial pressure or posttraumatic headache involve the entire head. Headaches related to sinus disease tend to focus over the sinuses. Temporomandibular joint pain, which may spread to involve the hemicrania, usually begins in the temporomandibular joint and is related to use of that structure, such as chewing.

Precipitating factors are important to understand. Migraines are often triggered by foods (Table 1). Headaches arising from osteoarthritis are more likely to be related to activity.

Clinicians should know if there is an aura that precedes the headache. Migraine is often signalled by some repetitive event that the patient comes to recognize. Precipitating and aggravating factors are important to identify. For example, migraines are usually related to minor stresses or food intake, temporomandibular joint pain is commonly precipitated by eating, while cervical headaches are more likely to be related to physical activities. Factors that relieve the headache must also be identified. A headache that is relieved by rest or medication is less likely to be related to intracranial disease than is one that persists despite physical activity and mild analgesics. It is important to examine the patient's level of psychosocial stress. While there are many named headache syndromes, most patients have nondescript headaches that are likely to be related to stress. A history of head trauma certainly raises the strong possibility of posttraumatic headache. Many patients have a family history of headaches, particularly migraines, which is helpful in establishing the diagnosis.[6,7]

Physical Examination

The general physical examination is rarely helpful,[5] although some specific abnormalities may be found. For example, evidence of oromandibular dysfunction includes the jaw opening

Table 1: Migraine Headache Prevention Program

Foods to avoid

Caffeine	Coffee, tea, iced tea, and cola; taper over 2 weeks, then *none*; decaffeinated versions are generally acceptable, although decaffeinated coffee and tea may be a problem for some people
Chocolate	
Cheese	Avoid all cheeses except American, cream, and cottage cheese. Avoid cheese-containing foods such as pizza
Monosodium glutamate	Chinese restaurant food, many snack and prepared foods, and seasoning products; MSG may be labelled as hydrolyzed vegetable/soy/plant protein, natural flavorings, yeast extract, Kombu, "broth," "stock," and others; *read labels*
Yogurt and sour cream	
Nuts	Including peanut butter
Processed meats	Those that are aged, canned, cured, marinated, tenderized, or contain nitrates or nitrites, including hot dogs, sausage, bacon, salami, and bologna
Alcohol and vinegar	Especially red wine, champagne, and dark or heavy drinks; vodka is best tolerated; white vinegar is acceptable
Citrus fruits and juices	Oranges, grapefruits, lemons, limes, and pineapples, and their juices; vitamin C and citric acid are acceptable

(continued on next page)

Table 1: Migraine Headache Prevention Program *(continued)*

Other fruits	Bananas, raisins, red plums, canned figs, and avocados
Certain vegetables	Lima, fava, navy, and broad beans; pea pods, sauerkraut, and onions
Certain bread products	Fresh-baked, yeast-risen bread products—such as from a bakery, doughnut shop, or home

Aspartame (Nutrasweet®)

Medications to avoid

Caffeine-containing medications	Excedrin®, Anacin®, Fiorinal®, Fioricet®, etc.
Sinus/decongestant medications	Actifed®, Dimetapp®, Dristan®, Sine-Aid®, Sudafed®, nasal sprays, and all other sinus and cold products that contain decongestants; plain antihistamines (such as Chlor-Trimeton®) *without* decongestants are acceptable; check with your pharmacist

Notes: This migraine headache prevention program may not be fully effective until you have been on it for at least 1 month. Caffeine withdrawal may be associated with temporarily increased headaches. In some cases, this dietary program alone may never adequately control migraine symptoms. In such cases the addition of migraine-preventive medicine may be advisable.
Even if you take migraine-preventive medication, you should follow this program. Without this program, migraine-preventive medication may not have an opportunity to work.
You should *strictly* follow this program until your migraine symptoms are adequately controlled. Then, you may wish to experiment with an item you have been avoiding, trying *one at a time* so that you can assess its individual effect on your symptoms. If eating or drinking an item is associated with recurrent symptoms, you should continue avoiding it.

Copyright © 1996 David Buchholz, MD

asymmetrically, an asymmetrical bite, or crepitus felt over the temporomandibular joints. Tenderness may be found in the suboccipital region. Cervical muscle spasm is common. With unilateral headache, be sure to palpate the superficial temporal artery. A unilateral enlarged and tender artery suggests temporal arteritis. Remember that these extracranial vessels become tender in migraine as well. Compress the sinuses, looking for acute or chronic sinus disease, and remember that the teeth are a common cause of head pain, although headache from dental disease is rare.

The neurologic examination should be normal. A careful cranial nerve evaluation is critical. Abnormalities suggest structural lesions of the brain or at the base of the skull. Listen to both carotid arteries for bruits. Palpate the superficial temporal arteries bilaterally, and be sure to listen for bruits in the vertebral system.

Headache as a symptom of cerebrovascular disease is quite common. Remember, hypertension is a common cause of headache. Look for papilledema, suggesting increase in cranial pressure, and perform a visual field examination to be certain there is no evidence of chiasmal compression.

The physical examination is usually more valuable for what it does not show than for abnormalities found. In most of the typical headache syndromes, no physical findings will be apparent.

Common Headache Syndromes

(1) *Migraine.* Migraine is probably the most common of all headache syndromes, except possibly for the muscular tension headache. Migraine headaches are usually unilateral and are often related to minor stresses or food intake. A list of the common foods that produce migraine is found in Table 1. Many patients have an aura warning that the migraine will occur. Typically, the migraine comes on shortly after awakening and progresses through the day. Most last 6 or 8 hours, many will last longer, and some persist for days. The first phase is characterized by aura and a vigorous pulsation in the external carotid system on the side of the headache. Most are in the distribution of the external carotid. Occasionally, a patient will have a posterior circulation migraine syndrome. In the second phase of the headache,

neurologic symptoms are common; these are usually visual, such as visual scotomata or visual hallucinations, but also include transient ischemic attacks. Occasionally, patients will suffer a migraine headache that does not relent, or repetitive headaches that come so rapidly there is virtually no time between them.

The typical headache can be relieved by sleep. Malaise and nausea often precede or accompany a migraine, and a euphoric period follows.

Treatment consists of dietary restrictions to avoid those foods that characteristically bring on headaches, when these foods can be identified for individual patients. Minor stresses often produce a headache. Many patients have noted that major stresses do not seem to cause headaches. Caffeine-containing compounds have been used for years to treat migraine. Ergot compounds (Ergomar®, Ergostat®, Wigrettes®) are used in the early phase to abort the period of vasodilation that characterizes the late stage of the headache. The approval of sumatriptan (Imitrex®) has provided dramatic improvement in the management of headache. Many patients can abort the headache at any phase by taking this drug. It is available by injection and in oral form. Begin with an oral dose of 25 mg or 50 mg. If this is effective, then the patient can simply be kept supplied with the medication. If it is not, try the injectable form, particularly if the headache is an uncommon event. Patients can be shown how to use the ready-packaged injection.

Patients with migraines can usually achieve satisfactory relief with a combination of strict diet and drug management. If these straightforward medications are not beneficial, consider referral to a headache specialist.

(2) *Tension headache.* The so-called tension headache is usually bitemporal and bilateral in the suboccipital region and clearly related to psychological stress. Some believe that underlying cervical spondylosis is the principal cause. In fact, patients who complain of headache from upper cervical discogenic disease and those who have stress-related tension headaches cannot be differentiated on the basis of the clinical features of their syndrome.

Tension headache is stereotypical, spreads in the distribution of C2 and C3 bilaterally, and is also felt in the bitemporal and bifrontal regions. Patients often say the pain feels as if a band is strapped around their heads. Sometimes the association with cervical disease is obvious. Sometimes there is no evidence of cervical disease. Some experts do not believe that cervical arthritis produces headache, while others believe that pain in the C2-3 distributions is typical, and that cervical spondylosis can cause typical tension headache.

If the cervical spine is suspected on the basis of spondylitic changes, treatment includes cervical traction, isometric exercises to strengthen cervical musculature, and local treatment for myositis and spasm. Relief of tension is important when the headaches are stress related. Mild analgesics (Motrin®) and antianxiety agents (Vistaril®) are both useful.

The so-called *tension-like headaches* are characteristically associated with both minor and major stresses in the patient's life. Teaching the patient to deal with these stresses may be useful. Biofeedback, psychological counseling, and other forms of stress therapy are commonly used. Mild antianxiety agents may be useful, but all of them have some habituation properties and may cause withdrawal symptoms. Cervical headaches can be alleviated by active physical therapy, such as traction and collar use, and by local physical therapy measures, such as triggerpoint injection, heat, cold, and TENS.[6]

(3) *Cluster headache.* This is similar to migraine, but is typically located in and around the eye.[8] The triggering factors are not as obvious as with migraine. Excessive eye watering and blurred vision may occur. Cluster headaches tend to be episodic, and there may be a seasonal variation, but this is still uncertain. Patients generally do not benefit from the typical migraine diet. Some patients who have what appear to be cluster headaches are improved substantially with sumatriptan, so this drug is worth trying. A number of surgical procedures have been developed for this syndrome. Some recommend microvascular decompression of the fifth cranial nerve, but clear benefits have not yet been reported. This type of headache is often associated with excessive sweating and lacrimation in the affected area. It it extremely dis-

abling to some patients, and a frustrating syndrome to treat. Unlike migraine, referral to a headache specialist is often necessary.

(4) Similar headaches that are poorly understood but are like migraine or cluster, are the so-called *ice cream headache* and the *exertional cough headache*. The ice cream headache is exactly what the name implies: a hemicranial headache indistinguishable from migraine that is characterisically set off by eating ice cream or other cold substances. The exertional cough headache is similar, but is brought on spontaneously by coughing. These and other similarly odd headaches have been reported rarely and are poorly understood. Treatment remains symptomatic and begins with avoidance.

(5) *Headache associated with head trauma* is particularly difficult. Many patients who have minor head trauma complain of persistent headache after recovery. The cause of the headache is unknown. The headache appears to be constant, although it can be worsened by emotional stress. It often requires long-term analgesics for control. Remember, some patients may develop posttraumatic hydrocephalus, and this must always be considered, although it is rarely found. Treatment is symptomatic.

(6) *Headache associated with vascular disease.* Patients with carotid stenosis and intracranial or extracranial disease of the carotid arteries characteristically complain of headache. The headache is nondescript and usually involves the entire head, not the distribution of the abnormal vessels. The headache is typically constant, worsened when blood pressure is elevated, and not necessarily associated with any neurologic phenomenon.

(7) *Headache from intracranial disease.* The typical headache related to tumor, infection, or hydrocephalus is constant and usually severe. These are its distinguishing features. The headache is not relieved by simple measures. Anything that increases intracranial pressure, such as laughing, sneezing, or coughing, will aggravate the headache. The headaches are usually worse at night, and when reclining. If the problem is intracranial, such as a tumor or hydrocephalus, the patient will typically say it feels as if his or her head "is going to explode."

(8) *Headache from almost any disease that affects the head or upper neck.* Headaches are common when patients have visu-

al abnormalities, even something as simple as refractive errors. Head pain certainly occurs with upper cervical disease, with sinusitis, with infiltrative tumors anywhere in the skull or upper cervical spine, and with dental disease. Most of these pains are more focal, but any persisting pain that does not respond to simple measures should lead to an imaging study.

Remember that headache is a common symptom that does not necessarily suggest abnormalities of the head and neck. Headaches commonly occur as a withdrawal phenomenon. Patients who have been taking narcotics or imbibing significant quantities of alcohol may have severe headache during withdrawal. Headache is common with systemic infection and with systemic illness and may arise from psychological factors and stress. These headaches are generally bilateral, suboccipital, and bitemporal. Patients often describe a band-like pain.

Imaging the Patient With Headache

One of the major questions in patients with headache is when to employ imaging studies. In general, if the patient has a typical migraine, cluster, or tension headache, imaging is not necessary before therapy is begun. In unusual situations, it is reasonable to image early. But for typical headaches, only use imaging for those patients who do not respond to treatment. Focal head pain, constant headache unrelieved by simple measures, the presence of atypical neurologic abnormalities not usually associated with a headache syndrome, and failure to achieve relief of seemingly typical headaches are major indications for imaging. But the yield of imaging in patients with headache is extremely small. There is no reason to image most of these patients, and certainly not before routine therapies are used.

Treatment of Headache

The treatment of headache can be divided into two separate areas: the management of the acute headache and prophylaxis for chronic headache.

The rules for the acute headache are similar to those discussed in the management of most pain syndromes. Begin with simple nonnarcotics to see if they are effective. The NSAIDs are often beneficial and should be used first. Aspirin remains the most common drug taken for headache. When the headache is more severe, the use of opioids, such as codeine (Empirin®, Tylenol® with Codeine) or oxycodone (Percocet®, Roxicet™, Tylox®), is reasonable, as long as constant use is not required. For the severe episodic headache, parenteral narcotics may occasionally be required. For migraine, sumatriptan (Imitrex®) has become the standard and its oral or parenteral formulation will abort most headaches. The standard treatment for many years was ergot, and many different preparations are available. However, sumatriptan appears to be superior for most patients and now is the first-line treatment.

Remember that all these headache syndromes have a tendency to produce nausea, as do many of the medications, so a concomitant antinausea drug may be required.

For the prophylaxis of chronic headaches, several choices are available. Experts use the NSAIDs commonly. Ergot-containing compounds are also given regularly. Experts also use beta-adrenergic agonists and calcium channel-blocking agents. However, the effectiveness of sumatriptan in blocking a headache is reducing the use of all these chronic medications.

There is strong evidence that following a strict antimigraine diet is better than chronic medication use, and most patients can be managed satisfactorily with diet and occasional acute medication for breakthrough headache.

The treatment of cluster headache is a particular problem. Some patients respond to low doses of corticosteroids. Lithium carbonate is sometimes used. Many patients can abort the headache by inhaled oxygen, and some respond to intranasal local anesthetics. Some patients with cluster headaches have found that sumatriptan is also effective for them, and it has become my first-line choice. Nevertheless, cluster headache has become a difficult problem to treat and one that often requires referral to a headache expert. This is in contrast to migraine, where only a minority of patients are not controlled relatively easily with diet and sumatriptan.

References

1. Raskin NH: Facial pain. In: *Headache*. 2nd ed. New York, Churchill Livingstone, 1988, pp 333-373.

2. Bell WE: *Orofacial Pains: Classification, Diagnosis, Management*. 4th ed. Chicago, Year Book Publishers, 1989.

3. Loeser JD: Tic douloureux and atypical face pain. In: Wall PD, Melzack R, eds. *Textbook of Pain*. 2nd ed. Edinburgh, Churchill Livingstone, 1989, pp 535-543.

4. Sharav Y: Orofacial pain. In: Wall PD, Melzack R, eds. *Textbook of Pain*. 2nd ed. Edinburgh, Churchill Livingstone, 1989, pp 441-454.

5. Headache Classification Committee of the International Headache Society: Classification and diagnostic criteria for headache disorders, cranial neuralgias and facial pain. *Cephalalgia* 1988;9(suppl 7):12-96.

6. Adler CS, Adler SM, Packard RC: *Psychiatric Aspects of Headache*. Baltimore, Williams and Wilkins, 1987.

7. Olesen J, Edvinsson L, eds: *Basic Mechanisms of Headache*. Amsterdam, Elsevier, 1988.

8. Kudrow L: *Cluster Headache. Mechanisms and Treatment*. Oxford, Oxford University Press, 1980.

Chapter 8

Pain in Children

Pain In Neonates

There is an old, erroneous belief among physicians and nurses that neonates do not feel pain and, therefore, do not need pain treatment.[1] All evidence indicates that this concept is untrue. What is true is that the management of pain in neonates is more difficult than in older children because of neonates' inability to describe their pain and because of their higher risk for respiratory depression from narcotics. Consequently, children with potentially painful diseases should be treated with the same analgesics that are used in adults. The skilled physician or nurse should be alert to recognize the signs of pain in neonates (Table 1), such as elevated pulse, elevated blood pressure, and rapid breathing. Analgesics appropriate to the disease should be used whenever needed.[2,3]

Pain in Older Children

Pain complicates many diseases in pediatric patients. Children undergoing surgery and those with neoplastic disease can expect to experience the same pain that adults would suffer. The principles of pain management for children are the same as for adults. All that needs to be modified is the appropriate dose of drug.[4]

Fear of the unknown, being left alone, and the new experience of pain all compound the child's pain experience. There-

Table 1: Signs of Pain in Neonates

- elevated pulse
- crying
- elevated blood pressure
- agitation
- rapid breathing

fore, remember that the child's pain can be substantially reduced by education and by familiarizing the child with the hospital and hospital routine. Furthermore, the child's pain can be modified by parents, family, and friends. Family support can be all important. Substitutes for family members who are trained to gain the child's confidence, such as nurses and other caregivers on the wards, can greatly alleviate the child's suffering by reducing anxiety and providing comfort.

Chronic Pain Syndrome in Children

Some children are beset with chronic pain, but this syndrome is different from the chronic pain syndrome in adults. These chronic pain syndromes can equally incapacitate adults and children, who often are unable to go to school or participate in any family activities. However, among children, depression, anxiety, and drug misuse are rare. Headache, myofascial syndrome, and specific joint pains, particularly in the legs, are the most common complaints. No physical findings or underlying cause can be found. Careful psychosocial exploration often reveals a major conflict between parent and child, usually the mother. The syndrome is more common in young females, although both sexes are involved. Treatment depends on a thorough evaluation for an organic pain syndrome, careful psychosocial evaluation, and a therapy program that restores the child to function and resolves family conflicts.[4]

References

1. Kaplan DW, ed: Pediatric pain: diagnosis, assessment and management. *Pediatrician* 1989;16:1-124.

2. McGrath PA: *Pain in Children: Nature, Assessment and Treatment.* New York, Guilford Press, 1990.

3. McGrath PJ, Unruh A: *Pain in Children and Adolescents*. Amsterdam, Elsevier Science Publishers, 1987.

4. Schecter NL, ed. Acute pain in children. *Pediatr Clin North Am* 1989;36:781-1047.

Chapter 9

Miscellaneous Pain States

AIDS-Related Pain

P ain is one of the most common complaints of patients with AIDS,[1] estimated to occur in more than 90% of these patients. Pain in AIDS, which may be nociceptive or neuropathic (Table 1), is second only to fever as a reason for hospitalization.

Typical nociceptive pain states include dysphagia with esophageal spasms, oral and esophageal ulcers, nonspecific abdominal pain, biliary tract pain, pancreatitis, and bowel obstruction. These gastrointestinal events occur in 25% of patients. Esophageal pain is common and may be so severe that it prevents swallowing. Remember that gastrointestinal pain may be secondary to infection, typically *Candida albicans*, herpes simplex, cytomegalovirus, tuberculosis, or *Cryptosporidium*. It is important to treat the underlying disease, but pain is often not relieved, even with what is considered adequate treatment.

AIDS patients characteristically have nonspecific arthralgias and HIV-associated arthritis. Septic arthritis must be differentiated from these nonspecific varieties. It is easy to mistake polyarthralgias for mononucleosis. The pain and inflammatory changes characteristically involve large joints, are severe, and are migratory as well as intermittent. Unfortunately, most of these patients do not respond to nonsteroidal anti-inflammatory drugs (NSAIDs).

Nonspecific myopathies also occur. They may be inflammatory or noninflammatory. Toxic myopathy occurs, particularly after AZT (Retrovir®) use. A diffuse polymyositis is the most common syndrome. The typical complaints include muscle pain in many places of the body, usually worsened by activity.

Headache suggests intracranial inflammatory disease or neoplasm. Remember that treatment with AZT induces a nonspecific headache syndrome that may be difficult to differentiate from the headache of increased intracranial pressure. Many AIDS patients have brain tumors. Diffuse headaches *inside* the skull are common. Headache is an indication for imaging.

Long-acting narcotics (MS Contin®, Oramorph SR™) are the most appropriate treatment for most of the nociceptive pain states. Long-acting neural narcotics or the transdermal fentanyl patches (Duragesic®) are particularly effective.

Neuropathic pain is also common. Patients have sensory neuropathies that present characteristically with pain and paresthesias in hands and feet. They may be spontaneous, but commonly follow treatment. Postherpetic neuralgia occurs with increased frequency in AIDS patients (see Chapter 6).

As with other neuropathic pain states, treatment with tricyclic antidepressants, anticonvulsants, and membrane-stabilizing drugs are more useful than narcotics.

Because many AIDS patients have a history of intravenous drug abuse, it might be expected that they would require larger doses of narcotics for pain control. This has not proved to be the case. It appears that these patients have approximately the same pain complaints as the general population of AIDS patients and do not require more analgesics for pain relief.

Treatment of Burn-Related Pain

Virtually all serious burns produce severe, prolonged pain.[2] In addition to the ongoing severe pain of the burn itself, these patients are subject to short bouts of much more severe pain associated with cervical intervention, dressing change, wound cleansing, and hydrotherapy. Burn patients also have a higher incidence of sympathetically maintained pain, myofascial pain

Table 1: AIDS-related Pain States

Gastrointestinal

Adverse GI events occur in up to 25% of patients.

- Dysphagia
- Odynophagia
- Esophagospasm (esophageal pain, in particular, is significant and causes considerable discomfort because pain occurs every time a patient swallows)
- Esophageal/aphthous ulcers
- Nonspecific abdominal pain (GI pain may be idiopathic, treatment-related, or caused by one or more organisms, including *C albicans,* herpes simplex virus, cytomegalovirus, *Cryptosporidium,* or *Mycobacterium tuberculosis.* Treatment of the underlying disorder may or may not eliminate the pain.)
- Biliary tract disorders
- Pancreatitis
- Obstruction

Headache

- HIV-related (includes meningitis, encephalitis, and neoplasm)
- Non-HIV-related (includes migraine [≈30%] and tension [≈60%-70%])
- Iatrogenic (AZT-induced)

Neuropathies

- Symmetrical sensory neuropathies (The sensory neuropathies occur most frequently, presenting as pain in and/or paresthesias of the soles or fingers. They generally occur as toxic manifestations of AIDS treatment. Decreased ankle reflexes are also seen.)
- Inflammatory demyelinating polyneuropathies
    - Guillain-Barré syndrome
    - Mononeuritis multiplex
- Polyradiculopathy
- Postherpetic neuralgia

(continued on next page)

Table 1: AIDS-related Pain States *(continued)*

Rheumatologic

- Reactive arthritis (Reiter's syndrome; in reactive arthritis, patients present with severe joint symptoms unresponsive to NSAIDs)
- Nonspecific arthralgia (Nonspecific polyarthralgias are associated with a mononucleosis-like syndrome. Pain is generally severe, intermittent, and involves the large joints.)
- Psoriatic arthritis
- HIV-associated rthritis
- Septic arthritis

Myopathies/Myositis

Polymyositis and noninflammatory myopathies may manifest early in the disease; toxic myopathies occur later as a consequence of AZT use.

- Polymyositis (most common)
- Noninflammatory myopathy
- Pyomyositis
- Toxic myopathy/myositis

secondary to immobilization, and peculiar denervation pain related to cutaneous injury.

The first issue with severe burn is to bring the acute pain under control (Table 2). In most burn units, immediate control is sought with opioids sometimes supplemented by benzodiazepines given by intravenous infusion. These patients often are intubated and require intensive care in the first few days. The intramuscular absorption may be unpredictable, and even finding a place to give an injection can be difficult.

With less severe burns, long-acting oral narcotics may suffice, but IV infusion is preferable, particularly if the patient is able to personally control the infusion.

The additional pain brought on by procedures or surgery requires standard perioperative, peri-injury management. Severely painful procedures should be carried out under anesthesia. For

Table 2: Pharmacotherapy for the Burn Patient

General Considerations
- Wide variations in analgesic requirements exist among burn victims
- Pharmacokinetics and pharmacodynamics may be altered:
  - Cardiovascular and respiratory instability immediately postinjury
  - Almost universal presence of hypotension and vasodilatation with or without sepsis
- Patient may be intubated, splinted, or otherwise unable to articulate pain

Opioid/Benzodiazepine Infusion
- Indicated primarily for large burn injuries; may be used in mild-to-moderate burns in patients with severe pain
- Opioid infusions are used more safely in burn unit than on regular ward because of close supervision by nursing staff

Patient-Controlled Analgesia (PCA)
- Used successfully in adults and children for procedure-related pain
- Systems can be developed allowing patients to activate PCA with their lower extremities if there are upper-extremity burns

Nonopioid Analgesics (NSAIDs)
- NSAID use is controversial because of the risk of excessive bleeding and occurrence of GI problems

(continued on next page)

less painful procedures, be sure the medication is given far enough in advance to provide an adequate level of analgesia for the duration of the procedure and the time after the procedure when the pain can be expected to be more severe. Long-acting oral narcotics provide an excellent way to achieve this.

Table 2: Pharmacotherapy for the Burn Patient *(continued)*

Oral Opioids

- Opioids are generally first-line analgesics, titrated to cardiorespiratory stability
- Continuous monitoring required:
  - Neurologic status after limb injury
  - Neurovascular status after limb injury
- High, around-the-clock dosing usually needed

Noninvasive Drug Delivery Systems

- There are no completed studies of transdermal fentanyl in burn patients; its use is contraindicated in children
- Oral transmucosal fentanyl citrate preparations (the so-called fentanyl lollipop) are indicated for analgesia and sedation in both adults and children

Badly burned children are a special problem. There is a tendency to deny analgesics to children. The opioids are adequate, but there is evidence that morphine half-life is shortened and clearance increased in acutely burned children. For these reasons, patient-controlled analgesia has been used successfully in older children and their parents.

A special problem with burned patients, both adults and children, is cardiovascular and respiratory instability that may occur in the acute postburn phase. It is important that pain therapy does not accentuate these problems. Another problem is hypotension secondary to vasodilatation. The same considerations apply. Finally, many patients are intubated and not able to voice their pain complaints, which all too often means that consideration of pain is ignored by a staff concerned with lifesaving measures.

As with any other acute injury, oral narcotics are an excellent choice for pain relief. However, NSAIDs should not be used in burn pain because of the risk of gastrointestinal hemorrhage. If oral narcotics cannot be used, then IV infusion is the next best choice. Oral transmucosal fentanyl preparations are available for both adults and children and may be useful.

Interstitial Cystitis

This is a common problem that occurs almost exclusively in females of age 40 or below. Symptoms suggest a urinary tract infection, but no bacteria can be cultured. Patients typically complain of extreme urgency and frequency, which may lead to multiple voidings each hour. Suprapubic pain is constant. The etiology is unknown. The term cystitis suggests that it is an inflammatory disease but the evidence for this is not strong. Different explanations have been hypothesized, but none has found favor with most urologists. Because the cause is unknown, it is not surprising that treatment is nonspecific. A major goal must be pain relief.

Treatments are generally medical or local and mechanical. The principal medical therapies are tricyclic antidepressants and opioids. Distention of the bladder from repeated lavage is common, but often makes the pain worse. Intravesical treatment with dimethyl sulfoxide (Rimso®-50) is used.

As is often the case with a nonspecific syndrome, there is debate about the influence of psychological factors. Obviously, patients with nonspecific complaints must also be evaluated for the possibility of primary or concurrent psychiatric disease. Nonspecific pain complaints are also common among drug seekers.

Chronic Pelvic Pain in Women

Chronic pelvic pain is a common problem. An estimated 10% of all visits to a gynecologist involve a complaint of unexplained pelvic pain.

The possible causes are heterogeneous and numerous, including endometriosis, dysmenorrhea, vaginismus, pelvic myofascial pain, local inflammation, interstitial cystitis, and pelvic neuropathies. Remember that entrapment syndromes involving the pudendal, ilioinguinal, iliohypogastric, and genitofemoral nerves may all occur. Unfortunately, one of the largest categories is idiopathic, with no clear etiology ever being discovered.[3]

Even when no obvious cause is found, a hysterectomy is sometimes performed. It is common for the pelvic pain to be considered psychological in origin.

Characteristically, patients with chronic pelvic pain experience multiple referrals and are transferred between medical specialties and among specialists.

Diagnosis of Chronic Pelvic Pain. All such patients should have an expert pelvic examination. Pelvic imaging, including both MRI and CT, will demonstrate many abnormalities. Endoscopic evaluation of the pelvis is now possible and allows accurate diagnosis when imaging studies are not definitive. Pelvic neuropathies are suggested when pain is limited to the distribution of a specific nerve and can be relieved by proximal blockade of that nerve. Often a trigger point suggesting a neuroma or area of compression can be found by palpation.

Psychological Factors in Chronic Pelvic Pain. Psychological factors appear to be important, although their impact in chronic pelvic pain syndrome is uncertain and remains controversial. However, many physicians think the comorbidities are important in either the genesis or the maintenance of the pain. Some 20% to 30% of women with chronic pelvic pain have experienced childhood abuse, and the incidence is much higher in patients with idiopathic pain. In these patients, chronic pelvic pain is considered a form of posttraumatic stress disorder. Patients with chronic pelvic pain are also said to have a higher incidence of somatization disorders. It is not clear that the somatization preceded the pain complaint. Women with chronic pelvic pain exhibit secondary depression, anxiety disorders, and substance misuse or abuse, as do other patients with developing chronic pain syndrome. Whether these problems are reactions to the pain or a part of the primary syndrome is a question that continues without resolution. Most agree that chronic pelvic pain is rare as a symptom of psychiatric disease or as a true conversion reaction. In contrast with other patients in the chronic pain syndrome, borderline personality and sociopathy appear to be rare.

These patients consistently exhibit sexual dysfunction. Most have pain after intercourse, many complain that sexual frequency is decreased, and they have a concomitant decrease in desire. These sexual problems consistently have negative effects on the marriage or relationship of these patients. Psychological factors are complex, but include loss of femininity, feelings of inadequacy, and guilt over failing to reproduce. The relationship with sexual partners becomes complex. At first, partners tend to be supportive, but with time they become less and less supportive. The patient is often accused of faking pelvic pain to avoid sex.

Typically, patients who exhaust symptomatic therapeutic alternatives are left with three options: (1) accept the fact that the pain is psychological and begin psychiatric treatment; (2) undergo surgical removal of organs that are apparently painful; or (3) learn to live with the pain.

Evaluation and Treatment of Chronic Pelvic Pain. Evaluation should begin with a thorough gynecologic examination by an expert. Then imaging studies should be used according to the expert's guidance. Diagnostic blocks may be helpful if an entrapment neuropathy is suspected. Because of the concomitant psychological issues, a skilled psychiatric assessment is usually worthwhile, particularly if no obvious cause of the problem is found. Treatment should first be directed at specific abnormalities. Arbitrary removal of pelvic organs without clear demonstration of disease is rarely worthwhile. Treatment of comorbidity, such as anxiety and depression, is important. The medications used for neuropathic pain (see Chapter 6) are often helpful. If explanations are not found promptly, these patients can often benefit from referral to a multidisciplinary chronic pain treatment center, which has a focus on pelvic pain. The number of experts available is not large, and these problems are so specialized that referral to an expert in questionable cases is usually worthwhile.

References

1. O'Neill WM, Sherrard JS: Pain in human immunodeficiency virus disease: a review. *Pain* 1993;54:3-14.

2. Choinière M, Melzack R, Rondeau J, et al: The pain of burns: characteristics and correlates. *J Trauma* 1989;29:1531-1539.

3. Hanno PM: Interstitial cystitis: when should you suspect it? what can you do about it? *Emerg Med* June 15, 1989:149-161.

Chapter 10

Appropriate Use of Narcotics in Severe Pain

M uch misunderstanding exists about the appropriate use of narcotics in patients with severe pain. When considering prescribing narcotics, clinicians must weigh a number of variables: (1) Nonnarcotic analgesics generally are not effective enough to relieve severe pain. (2) Many patients complain of severe pain for which no obvious cause can be found and profess to be completely disabled by it. Misuse of narcotic analgesics by these patients is common, that is, many of them take narcotics in quantities that exceed doses usually prescribed for relief of serious pain. (3) While misuse is much more common than frank addiction, drug-seeking behavior with regard to prescription drugs certainly does occur. (4) The long-term effects of narcotics are not well known. (5) The patient in severe pain does not have many medical alternatives other than narcotics. (6) The prescription of narcotics is controlled by regulations of state and federal agencies, which can impose serious penalties for inappropriate prescribing.

For all of these reasons, it is important to understand current thought on the appropriate use of narcotics for pain relief and to follow a uniform personal policy. It is equally important to understand that this is a field in which concepts are changing. New drugs and more information about long-term narcotic use will become available. These guidelines must be continually updated for maximum efficacy.

Narcotic Use For Cancer Pain

Described in detail in Chapter 4, the basic principles of narcotic use in cancer patients are these. First, establish a diagnosis and understand the cause of the pain. Treat the underlying condition, whether cancer or some complicating issue. Use nonnarcotic analgesics as a first step. If they are ineffective, move to the lesser narcotics such as oxycodone (Percodan®, Roxicodone™) and codeine (Empirin® with Codeine, Tylenol® with Codeine). As these become less effective, use long-acting oral narcotics such as methadone (Dolophine®), morphine (MS Contin®, Oramorph SR™), or transdermal fentanyl (Duragesic®). Remember to treat anxiety and depression.

As long as the patient is mentally alert and does not have systemic side effects, the actual dose of narcotic can vary, but the goal is pain control without the side effects that diminish the patient's quality of life. If adequate analgesia cannot be obtained with reasonable doses of narcotics, anxiety and depression may be playing an important role in the pain syndrome. If the patient is not satisfactorily relieved with tolerated doses of narcotics, then the clinician must look for expert help to define and treat the problem.[1]

Narcotic Use After Acute Injury

The goal of analgesics after acute injury is patient comfort. The patient should be given narcotics in doses adequate to relieve pain if nonnarcotic analgesics do not provide sufficient pain relief. Parenteral drugs should be used for acute pain after serious injury or operation, typically for about 48 to 72 hours. Generally, oral narcotics are not as effective as the parenteral forms because the doses used are not equipotential. Therefore, the patient does not achieve adequate relief. Another common problem with oral agents is administering the drugs at intervals that do not relate to their duration of action. Whatever oral drug is used should be given in doses expected to provide analgesia equivalent to what the patient requires parenterally. Oral drugs should be given on a schedule that relates to their duration of action, not to some ill-defined plan to limit their intake. It makes no sense to give a drug every 6 hours when its expected analgesia will only last 3 hours. The common error I see is an attempt to switch from adequate parenteral analgesia to substantially smaller amounts of oral narcotics and at intervals of 6 hours.

Evidence indicates that postoperative and serious postinjury pain require substantial analgesic use in the first 48 hours. We should then expect a steady decline in amount of drug and frequency of dose. Most patients rarely use narcotic analgesics after the fifth postoperative or postinjury day. Some operations that are known to be more painful require substantial analgesia for longer periods. Most patients do not need narcotics after the second week. Patients who require narcotics longer than this for supposed incisional pain may have a painful complication or may be exhibiting drug-seeking behavior. It is important to determine which.

While inadequate analgesia after surgery or injury is the most common error in analgesic use, prolonged inappropriate use of analgesics is still an issue. Some patients, often without a history of illicit or prescription drug use, persist in their request for narcotics weeks to months after surgery or injury. Because we cannot know what these patients experience or what benefits they receive from the narcotic, it is difficult to deal with these issues on an individual basis. My rules about their management are simple. Two to 4 weeks of narcotic analgesia postsurgery are adequate even for most serious and pain-producing procedures. Incisional pain persisting longer than this should be considered suspicious and the patient should be evaluated to be certain that a pain-producing complication does not exist. Incisional pain should not require narcotics indefinitely after healing.

A similar problem exists when postoperative or postinjury patients use quantities of narcotics substantially greater than those typically prescribed. While patients vary according to age and size, these variations require only small adjustments in dose. Patients should not be allowed to use narcotic doses substantially greater than those expected to provide adequate analgesia, nor given narcotics for longer than the expected duration of pain with the specific injury.[2]

Use of Narcotics in Chronic Severe Pain of Benign Origin

The use of narcotics in managing patients who complain of intractable pain of benign origin is a complex issue. To understand the evolution of current practice, we must go back to the emergence of pain management as a subspecialty in medicine in the 1960s. Our experience in The Johns Hopkins Pain Treatment Center is typical and a review of that experience will aid in understanding the situation today.[2]

As patients complaining of pain were admitted to pain treatment centers, it was obvious to all of those involved in therapy that there were substantial comorbidities in addition to the medical problem of pain. The most important of these comorbidities were psychiatric disorders.

Approximately 15% of patients suffered from easily diagnosed psychiatric disease in which pain was a major complaint. These patients virtually never had an obvious cause of pain or a diagnosis competent to produce the pain. We concluded that, in these patients, pain was the symptom of the psychiatric disease. Approximately 30% of patients had no evidence of primary or endogenous psychological dysfunction, although many were secondarily depressed. The remainder were found to have personality dysfunction antedating their pain problem and were disabled beyond the levels expected on the basis of diagnosis and physical impairments.

Reactive depression and anxiety were present in all three groups, although less obvious in those with psychiatric diagnoses.

Drug-use patterns were interesting. Only a minority of patients were not taking narcotic analgesics. True addiction with drug-seeking behavior was relatively infrequent (14%). However, nearly half were using narcotics at levels beyond those usually prescribed and the remainder were using narcotics at levels within the limits usually prescribed by physicians. The use of antianxiety agents, principally diazepam (Valium®), was similar.

Because drug misuse was such an important issue in most patients, mandatory withdrawal programs were started. About 10% of patients refused withdrawal and left the program, but the remainder were withdrawn successfully. The point of greatest interest is that in a group of nearly 500 patients withdrawn from oral short-acting narcotics, not one thought the pain was worse after withdrawal. However, nearly 10% thought their pain was substantially relieved. We, and most other pain experts, interpreted the evidence to conclude that patients with chronic pain did not benefit from short-acting oral narcotics and that drug-seeking behavior, overuse, and cognitive, as well as systemic, side effects were common. For these reasons, most experts in chronic pain ceased to use short-acting narcotic analgesics and insisted on withdrawal as part of a therapy program.

Long-Acting Oral Narcotics for Management of Chronic Pain

The development of effective oral narcotics reopened the question of whether narcotics should be used to relieve chronic pain of benign origin over long periods of time. From the purely medical standpoint, the answer to this question is simply not known. There are no good comparative studies, either efficacy studies or controlled trials, which demonstrate that narcotics are safe and effective when administered over many years. Critics of the idea, and those experienced with narcotics, contend that tolerance will be a limiting factor and that side effects may be substantial. There is little evidence that addiction to long-acting oral narcotics will be a concern, but the physiologic habituation with the potential for withdrawal is a real issue.[3]

With those reservations, it is reasonable to consider long-acting oral drugs for chronic pain of benign origin. Our current usage requires the following entrance criteria. There must be a defined medical problem competent to cause the pain of which the patient complains. Pain relief should be adequate to restore the patient to function. Pain relief should be accompanied by increased function when pain has been the cause of disability. There should be no long-term side effects on cognition. Periodic re-evaluation and assessment of both liver and kidney function are important. Patients are not allowed to escalate the dose.

Our experience has been instructive but leaves many questions unanswered. The first issue is pain control. Among my patients who have been treated in the specialized program we have organized to deal with long-term use of oral narcotics, I judge pain control to have been marginal. An occasional patient has dramatic relief, improved function, and meets all the criteria that we consider success. Most say pain relief is better, but not satisfactory, and do not improve either vocational or personal functions. Many patients develop unpleasant side effects, usually reduction in cognitive ability, and the drug must be discontinued. Drug-seeking behavior has not been an issue and patients who were difficult to manage when taking the short-acting oral narcotics do not exhibit the same focus on their medications. However, most of the patients who had drug abuse or misuse problems before using long-acting narcotic therapy claim that narcotics in this form are ineffective and discontinue the program promptly.

I reserve long-term oral narcotic therapy for those patients with clearly defined painful problems for which no additional treatment is possible. Depression and anxiety must be treated adequately and most patients are referred to a comprehensive pain treatment program for the therapies that would eliminate the need for narcotics in any form. I do not maintain any patients on short-acting oral narcotics.

If this route of pain management is considered, clinicians must be certain that the complaint of pain is not indiscriminately treated with narcotics. That was the error of 30 years ago. Patients with overt psychiatric disease and pain complaints as a part of that disease should receive appropriate psychiatric care. Patients whose psychosocial problems outweigh medical problems must also be evaluated and treated. In my experience, most have work disability claims based on the complaint of pain, not physical impairment. Most are disabled by back or neck pain. We have long experience in dealing with patients with significant spinal abnormalities. Their limitations, behaviors, and drug requirements are well known. Narcotic therapy is not indicated for back pain patients who have no significant spinal abnormality or who are disabled with spinal disease beyond anything reasonable. However, we must avoid the trap of believing that if we cannot make a diagnosis, no one can. Referral of such patients to experts is justified.

It is also important to avoid another common error. Many physicians believe that if they have not made a definitive diagnosis, then the patient's complaints are psychiatric in origin and the process is psychosomatic. Psychiatric diagnoses are made on positive signs and symptoms, just as are medical diagnoses. The absence of one does not diagnose the other.

When Is Narcotic Therapy Reasonable in Chronic Pain of Benign Origin?

No definitive answer exists to this question, and many more years of research are likely before general answers can be formulated. However, there are guidelines on which reasonable practice can be based. First, the patient should have a diagnosable medical problem known to cause severe pain. A complaint of pain is not enough. Desire for narcotics is not an adequate reason to prescribe them. Then, all reasonable therapies should have been exhausted. If the underlying problem can be treated by other means with reasonable certainty of success and at low risk, then narcotics should not be considered as an alternative. Treatments that are uncertain and/or of high risk should not be required prior to a decision for narcotic therapy. Patients should be informed of the consequences of therapy. They need to know that the outcome of long-term narcotic treatment is uncertain and that its long-term physiologic effects on them are not known. I tell patients that I consider the treatment investigational. Patients need to know details of all of the potential side effects and particularly must be warned about the impact on cognitive functions. Physicians must be prepared to follow the patient at regular intervals and examine physiologic functions periodically. Reasonable changes in narcotic use may be expected, but significant dose escalation is not acceptable.

Criteria for Success

The hallmark of success is pain relief. However, professed pain relief alone is not enough. When patients are disabled by pain, then pain relief should lead to improvements in vocational and personal function and to decreased use of medical resources. If none of these things occurs, then I do not consider the patient's claim of adequate pain relief as credible.

A successful program is also characterized by lack of escalation of dose, lack of drug-seeking behavior, and lack of important side effects.

Impediments to Long-Term Narcotic Use

While any licensed physician can prescribe narcotics, a number of impediments, both legal and psychological, must be managed. In many states, it is illegal for a physician to maintain an addict outside of a recognized program for treatment of addiction. You must be certain that an addict for whom you prescribe narcotics is, in fact, enrolled in a treatment program. Physician prescribing practices are monitored and aberrations will be reported often to state licensing agencies. Many states do not allow physicians to provide narcotics for themselves or for family members or in unusual quantities to patients. Therefore, when a patient is given long-term oral narcotics for pain control, it is critical that the reasons are clearly defined both in the medical record and to those who may be involved in surveillance. In our practice the decision for long-term narcotic maintenance is made by a pain expert, but the actual patient maintenance is carried out by someone else. Before choosing narcotic maintenance, it is usually wise to seek consultation with an expert in pain-producing disease for confirmation of diagnosis and affirmation of the treatment plan.

Psychological issues affect both physicians and patients. Most physicians do not understand the use of oral narcotics and are frightened by the large doses required. They and other health-care professionals look upon narcotic use as synonymous with addiction. Patients fear that use of narcotics may lead them to addiction, to illicit drugs, or to drug-seeking behavior. Some patients have the opposite view and do not seem to understand the potential dangers of the side effects of narcotics. If narcotics are used for the treatment of chronic pain, they must be employed within clear guidelines and with the understanding that harmful side effects not currently expected could appear with time. You must be prepared to modify guidelines as new data become available.

The Danger Signs

A series of patient actions strongly suggests addiction or misuse. Typically, patients want more and more drug, particularly short-acting narcotics or parenteral supplements for bouts of severe pain. Patients often want specific drugs and ask for them by name. They frequently excuse the need for more drug by stereotyped explanations. Among the most common are: *"the medication was stolen," "more is needed for a vacation," "the medicine was dropped in the toilet,"* or *"the medication was used by a family member."* There may be frequent trips to emergency rooms for additional medication based on complaints of severe exacerbations of pain. These patients often wait until the last possible moment for refills, and choose evenings, weekends, and holidays to call for more medication when they know the chances are best for receiving the medication without re-evaluation. Such patients commonly receive the same medication from several different physicians. The record holder among my patients was receiving the same medications from 14 physicians, all on the staff of the same hospital.[2]

Transdermal fentanyl seems to have little abuse potential and is a good choice for long-term therapy, particularly in patients with a history of drug misuse.

Remember, not all of these drugs are taken by the patient. Many are sold.

Any drug-seeking behavior is suspect and the patient should be evaluated by someone expert in the management of medical addiction. Drug misuse cannot be allowed. It endangers the patient and places at risk your ability to practice medicine.

Summary

Clinicians must learn well the characteristics of the narcotic medications they choose to use, understand the conversions between parenteral and oral narcotics, and use narcotics in appropriate doses for appropriate periods of time as indicated by the underlying disease. Clinicians should not prescribe narcotics for unexplained pain. Look for a cause and treat it. There is no reason why any patient with cancer or with an acute injury should suffer unnecessarily. Side effects should be considered the major limitation on narcotic use. Physiologic habituation is not a major issue. No patient should be treated excessively either in terms of the choice of narcotics or the length of administration. Tailor narcotic use to the natural history of the pain-producing process. Short-acting narcotics are virtually never indicated for long-term use. They are ineffective and the misuse/abuse potential is high. The use of long-acting oral narcotics for chronic pain of benign origin is still being investigated. It can be justified based on current information, provided specific guidelines are followed. If this route is chosen, it is always wise to have concurrence from another independent physician and the opinion of an expert in pain management. Be sure the patient understands that long-term side effects are not known and that systemic problems not yet appreciated may develop. There is no excuse for maintaining addiction or tolerating drug-seeking behavior. Patient insistence is not an excuse for poor medical practice.

The rational use of narcotics can greatly benefit patients and alleviate much suffering. Irrational use will potentially harm patients and cannot be excused.[3]

References

1. Foley KM: The treatment of cancer pain. *N Engl J Med* 1985; 313:84-95.

2. Long DM: Acute and chronic pain. In: Davis JH, Drucker WR, Foster RS, et al, eds. *Clinical Surgery*. Volume 1. St Louis, Missouri, CV Mosby Co, 1987, pp 509-534.

3. Payne R, Foley KM, eds: *The Medical Clinics of North America: Cancer Pain*. Philadelphia, WB Saunders Co, 1987.

///// Chapter 11

Surgery for Pain

The earliest surgery for the treatment of pain was in the late 1800s and entailed the division of individual nerves. Cutting posterior sensory roots became popular around the turn of this century. Division of the anterior spinothalamic tract became an option after the clinical observation that a patient with bilateral lesions in this area of the spinal cord did not feel pain below the abnormal level. As our understanding of the anatomy of the pain system increased, so did the number of attempts to interrupt the pain transmission at every accessible level. Most of these have been eliminated and the surgical procedures now used for pain are mostly nondestructive. Even the destructive procedures are generally less invasive than the direct surgical procedures of the earlier era.

Traditionally, surgery on the pain pathways has been presented anatomically, beginning in the periphery and proceeding centrally in the same sequence as the pain system transmits. That still is a convenient way to present the surgical procedures that are occasionally done for pain.[1,2]

Neurotomy

Cutting peripheral nerves is rarely indicated. However, in a few circumstances destruction of a painful peripheral nerve still may be useful. When a painful neuroma exists on a transected nerve, cutting the nerve proximal to the neuroma can be effective so that the next neuroma formed will not be easily traumatized. Some clinicians have advocated multiple nerve sections with re-anastomosis in an attempt to prevent neuroma formation. Rarely, nonessential nerves may be entrapped either naturally or in a surgical scar. Pain in the groin following inguinal hernia repair is a typical example. Identifying and cutting the entrapped nerve is reasonable treatment when nerve function can be sacrificed. Another typical condition that warrants neurotomy is the postthoracotomy syndrome, which produces intractable pain because of injury to an intercostal nerve. Identifying the nerve and sectioning it will usually cure the pain.

Open division of intercostal nerves has been replaced with percutaneous radiofrequency destruction. An appropriate needle electrode is introduced near the nerve and radiofrequency heat is used to destroy nerve function. Since pain fibers are smaller and thus more sensitive to heat, it is sometimes possible to eliminate pain sensation without significant injury to other sensations.

Another use of peripheral neurotomy is in the so-called facet denervation. The medial branch of the posterior primary ramus, which innervates the zygapophyseal joint, is identified as it crosses the lumbar transverse process and these nerves are destroyed by percutaneous radiofrequency. The resulting joint denervation often relieves back pain without any deleterious consequences.

The principles involved in choosing nerves for section are straightforward. The nerve in question is first anesthetized to determine pain relief. When temporary blockade produces satisfactory pain relief, then section of the same nerve in a similar location should produce lasting pain relief. The local anesthetic also allows the patient to experience the sensory loss and to determine if it is acceptable.

Posterior Rhizotomy

An alternative to section of peripheral nerve is division of the posterior sensory roots. This is particularly useful for pain involving the trunk where the loss of sensation is not important

144

It has also been useful for head and neck cancer. The operation is formidable because the spinal cord and/or brain stem must be exposed and the posterior roots individually sectioned. Some have advocated differential section of the laterally placed, pain-carrying sensory roots or individual sections in the spinal cord undercutting these lateral sensory roots where they enter the cord.

It is common to identify the roots to be sectioned by temporary blockade, usually at the neural foramen. This allows the patient to experience the sensory loss and helps the surgeon determine which roots need to be sectioned.

Neurotomy and rhizotomy have both been used for leg pain in the failed back syndrome. Success rates have not been high and few use either procedure now.

The principal use of posterior rhizotomy has been for head and neck cancer when coupled with division of the fifth cranial nerve.

Chemical Rhizotomy

Many patients who need rhizotomy are systemically ill from cancer and thus are not good candidates for major procedures. Destruction of posterior roots by intrathecal injection of neurolytic agents has been used in terminal patients. While it has been employed throughout the spinal axis, the most common technique involves destruction of lumbar and sacral roots for intractable pelvic pain of cancer. The procedure requires lumbar puncture for the instillation of absolute alcohol or phenol (usually about 4.5%). A contrast agent can be used so that the fluoroscopy can guide layering of the neurolytic agent to ensure that only posterior roots are injured.

Cordotomy

Section of the anterolateral spinothalamic tract produces analgesia on the body side opposite and below the cut. Section may be surgical (open) or percutaneous (radiofrequency). Cordotomies typically were carried out with a general anesthetic. The spinal cord was exposed and a knife used to cut the anterior quadrant, thus dividing the tract. Incisions were usually made at different levels to minimize neurologic deficit. Typically, one section would be made at C2 and the other at C5 or C6 for bilateral pain control. Alternatively, if pain relief was only needed in abdomen and lower extremities the incisions could be made in the upper thoracic region. In the early 1960s, open cordotomy was replaced by a percutaneous technique in which a fine needle was introduced into the spinal cord at C2 and a radiofrequency current was used to destroy the spinal cord. This percutaneous cordotomy is now the standard.

Pain control from cordotomy is excellent and the neurologic consequences of percutaneous cordotomy are not usually serious. Bilateral cordotomy has a much higher risk of significant neurologic deficit. The technique is now used principally for patients who have failed other measures. Cordotomy generally achieves complete analgesia on the side opposite the lesion. Because of the somatotopic relationship in the tract, some master surgeons have even been able to denervate specific parts of the body. The major complication is weakness on the side of the lesion.

Brain Stem Surgery for Pain

The pain tracts are also accessible in the brain stem and many surgeons have devised ways to cut them. But the consequences of brain stem incisions are generally greater than the benefits. Consequently, these techniques, whether done by open surgery or stereotactic methods, are little used today. Trigeminal descending root section is the most common technique in use.

Thalamic Surgery for Pain

Stereotactic surgeons have also attacked many targets in the thalamus, the most common being the principal sensory nuclei. As our understanding of the interconnections of the pain system in the thalamus increased, so did the number of targets. This remains a tool of experts for very specific reasons.

Cingulumotomy

The destruction of the cingulum as a kind of modified lobotomy for patients with intractable pain of cancer usually complicated by severe depression and anxiety was an effective technique. However, better ways to treat depression and anxiety and improved methods of pain control have virtually eliminated cingulomotomy except in unusual cases. The technique is stereotactic and requires destruction of the cingulum bilaterally as these fiber tracts course above the lateral ventricles. Personality consequences are minimal and pain relief is frequently satisfactory.

Neuroaugmentation or Stimulation of the Nervous System for Pain Control

In addition to the destructive techniques being used, stimulation of the nervous system has also been developed to control pain. Stimulation of the body as a means of relieving pain has a long history, going back several hundred years. The first electrical stimulation devices used electrodes attached to the skin. The sensory system was activated and pain relief sometimes followed. The transcutaneous electrical technique was developed in the hope of finding a screening procedure to predict benefit from one of the various forms of implantable nervous system stimulators developed in the late 1960s. These stimulators are small, fully implantable radiofrequency devices that are activated by a transcutaneous radio signal from an outside source. The radiofrequency signal is converted into an electrical signal, which in turn is applied to the nervous system, thus blocking pain. Stimulators have been developed for peripheral nerve, spinal cord, and brain.

Of these, only spinal cord stimulation is commonly used, usually for intractable pain of benign origin, such as for patients with failed back syndrome often complicated by arachnoiditis. Patients are chosen by testing their response to temporary stimulation. This is done by introducing an electrode into the epidural space above the area of pain and connecting it temporarily to an external stimulator. When this produces pain relief, the patient is a candidate for an implantable system.

The system consists of one of several kinds of electrodes available from the manufacturers. These are placed over the posterior aspect to the spinal cord. Some require direct surgical implantation, while some can be inserted percutaneously. They are positioned to provide stimulation that covers the painful area and then are attached to an internal receiver. Some of these devices have a permanently implanted battery source that is activated with external controls. In some, the radiofrequency generator is externally placed. Either way, patients have a control device to activate and deactivate at will, providing stimulation when pain control is required.

These devices are effective enough to become standard treatment for the patient with failed back syndrome who is not managed well by other means. Recent evidence suggests that the results may be as good as reoperation and may offer the patient an alternative to major reparative surgery. The major drawbacks are a small infection rate that requires removal of the device and electronic mechanical failures that occur with any implanted system.[2] Similar stimulating systems are available for peripheral nerves but are not often needed.

Deep brain stimulation has also been explored extensively. It is not now a standard technique, but is being examined by a few stereotactic surgeons. Stimulating electrodes are placed into the specific sensory nuclei of the thalamus or the reticular thalamic and periaqueductal gray areas that are thought to be related to the descending inhibitory system of pain. Brain stimulation is most commonly used for pain of nervous system origin. The outcomes reported by different surgeons have varied substantially. Overall, the technique has not proven successful enough to reach standard practice.

Trigeminal Neuralgia

Trigeminal neuralgia, or tic douloureux, is a specific problem for which surgery is commonly indicated. The clinical syndrome is typical. Patients have lancinating pain that occurs suddenly in the distribution of the trigeminal nerve. Typically, the pains have a trigger and can be brought on by touching, facial movement, swallowing, or even blinking. Patients often are unable to eat, shave, or brush their teeth. The pain is excruciating, but short lived. Some patients will have pain triggered so frequently that it seems almost continuous. There are no associated neurologic deficits. A similar syndrome may implicate tumors involving the trigeminal nerve. Brain-stem plaques from multiple sclerosis may produce the same clinical picture, often bilaterally.

The first treatment for trigeminal neuralgia is medical. Carbamazepine (Tegretol®) is the most effective drug. Administered in a dose of 200 to 800 mg/day, carbamazepine will relieve the tic pain in most patients. When confronted with a patient in tic crisis, the pain should be temporarily relieved by narcotics while carbamazepine is administered to a level that produces pain control. If the pain is not severe, begin with 200 mg/day and increase to 600 or 800 mg/day or until the pain is controlled. If the pain is severe, the larger dose should be given immediately and the patient should be warned of the side effect of somnolence. Pain relief should occur within a day or two and persist. Some patients are unable to tolerate the drug. Then phenytoin (Dilantin®) 100 to 300 mg/day can be substituted. If the patient is unable to tolerate either drug, surgical solutions are sufficiently effective so that intervention should not be withheld when medication is ineffective.

Chemical and Radiofrequency Rhizotomy

The procedure requires a brief general anesthetic. A needle is introduced into the cheek and then, with fluoroscopic control, guided through the foramen ovale into the gasserian ganglion. Two techniques are in common use. The first is injection of phenol into the ganglion. Some hypalgesia occurs and pain relief is usually immediate. Another technique is to enter the roots behind the ganglion with a fine-needle electrode and then use a radiofrequency technique to destroy these fibers. More sensory loss occurs, but the pain control usually lasts longer. Short-term success of these techniques is above 90% and usually lasts for some months. It may be permanent. Recurrence of pain is common, but the procedures are generally easy to repeat. Even elderly patients tolerate the procedures well.

Because of the recurrence rate, surgeons have continued to explore ways to provide more lasting relief without a permanent neurologic deficit. The original surgical techniques required avulsion of peripheral nerve branches, surgical section of the posterior root in the middle fossa, or surgical section of the posterior root in the posterior fossa. The resulting sensory loss is unpleasant. We now recognize that many patients with trigeminal neuralgia have apparently aberrant vessels compressing the posterior root in the posterior fossa. This has led to the development of so-called microvascular decompression. In the surgery, the posterior fossa trigeminal nerve is explored through a limited incision. Small vessels, either arteries or veins, are removed from the trigeminal root and kept away by appropriate packing. The success of the operation is remarkable. Recurrences do occur, but many patients achieve lasting relief.

The argument continues about which of these techniques is preferable for the treatment of trigeminal neuralgia. Microvascular decompression has a somewhat higher risk rate, but accomplishes lasting pain relief without neurologic deficit. The injection techniques are safer, somewhat less permanent, and have a small neurologic deficit associated with them.

My management philosophy is to use medication as long as it is satisfactory without unpleasant side effects. If the patient is elderly, I use the injection techniques because of safety. For younger patients, microvascular decompression offers a better chance at lasting relief. The choice of one initially does not preclude the subsequent use of another.

The acute crisis of intractable pain that occurs with trigeminal neuralgia is a medical emergency. These patients nearly always must be hospitalized, hydrated because they often cannot eat or drink, and they need immediate pain control. If narcotics are not effective, then urgent intervention should proceed to achieve pain control.

References

1. Gybels JM, Sweet WH: *Neurosurgical Treatment of Persistent Pain.* Basel, Karger, 1989.

2. Long DM: Surgical therapy of chronic pain. *Neurosurgery* 1980;6(3):317-328.

Chapter 12

Management of Neck Pain and Other Spinal Pain

N eck pain is one of the most common of all spinal syndromes, exceeded in incidence only by low back pain and headache. The syndromes that involve the nerve roots that make up the brachial plexus are specific and can be accurately localized. The syndromes of the upper cervical disks and axial pain are less well defined.

The causes of neck pain and of low back pain are similar and the fundamental concepts are the same. Degenerative disk disease is thought to be a cause of pain for both neck and low back, as is a dysfunctional segment. The structures are analogous and their potential to produce pain is the same.

History and Physical Examination in Cervical Pain

The first issue the clinician must address is the location of the pain. Is it only in the neck? Does it spread into the head, shoulders, or upper extremities? Where exactly is it located in the neck? Is it aggravated by activity and relieved by rest? Is it associated with loss of range of motion of the neck or with local muscular symptoms? As in the low back, spondylitic disease is generally worsened by activity and improved by rest. Focalized areas of muscle tenderness suggest myositis. The location of the pain and its radiation are important clues and will be described under the specific localizing syndromes.

The physical examination consists of inspection and palpation, looking for muscle spasm and trigger points. The patient's range of motion, flexion, extension, and rotation should be tested. Limitation of these functions suggests either arthritic disease or muscle spasm. Strength of shoulder girdle musculature and upper extremities and sensation from C1 to T1 should be tested. The reflexes of the upper extremities should be assessed and signs of myelopathy should be evaluated, such as hyperreflexia in the lower extremities or the presence of Hoffman's or Babinski's signs.

Specific Cervical Syndromes

Rotational movements of the head exacerbate pain at the cervical-occipital junction. This pain is specifically suboccipital and does not radiate.

Pain originating in the C1-2 articulation is suboccipital and radiates up the midline of the occipital region, but does not extend far enough laterally to involve the ear. Pain from the C2-3 articulation is also suboccipital, but extends laterally and may involve the ear. Aside from the suboccipital component, both of these sensations are perceived as head pain, rather than as neck pain.

Pain from the C3-4 area involves the midneck and midshoulders, but does not extend laterally over the shoulders. Pain from the C4-5 area is characteristically felt in the neck and radiates into the deltoid region laterally over the shoulders. Because of the innervation of the rhomboids by C5, there may be intrascapular radiation along the upper margin of the scapula. Weakness of deltoid function may occur. Abduction at the shoulder may be weak. If there is a sensory loss, it will usually be found over the outermost aspect of the shoulder and extend only slightly down over the lateral surface of the arm. Occasionally, biceps weakness may be present, but is not common.

Pain arising from the C5-6 space characteristically occurs in the midneck and radiates down the arm to the thumb and forefinger. It may be associated with weakness of the biceps. There may be a loss of both radioperiosteal reflex and biceps reflex.

Radiation may also occur to the inner scapular location at approximately its midpoint.

Pain arising from the C6-7 interspace characteristically occurs in the root of the neck and radiates down the posterior arm to the middle three fingers. There usually is not an associated motor loss. Sensory loss will involve some combination of the middle three fingers. Intrascapular pain occurs in the lower third of the scapula.

Pain arising from the C7-T1 space occurs in the root of the neck and radiates down the arm to the middle two fingers. Sensory loss is usually found in the 4th and 5th fingers. Weakness of intrinsic hand musculature may be present. The triceps reflex may be reduced with either C6-7 or C7-T1 disease. Subscapular radiation of pain is common.

Unfortunately, the syndromes are often not this specific; rather, patients complain of diffuse neck pain without specific radiations. However, it is worthwhile questioning them carefully because often the history of the pain will be adequate to localize the abnormality.

When the problem is simple disk herniation, the radicular component predominates. But this situation is relatively rare. Most patients complain of diffuse neck pain and do not have specific radicular complaints.

Imaging Studies

The principal imaging study is a series of plain x-rays that must include anterior-posterior and lateral films, oblique views to examine the foramina, and flexion/extension films to test for subluxation. Fractures, severe degenerative disease, and tumors will be demonstrated. However, for most patients, the findings will be nonspecific. Patients with severe degenerative disease do not necessarily have pain, so simply finding the degenerative disk disease does not guarantee that a cause of the pain has been discovered.

When the pain is only in the neck, plain x-rays are adequate to evaluate the patient initially. If there is a significant radicular component, it is probable that an additional imaging study will be required. Magnetic resonance imaging (MRI) is the study of choice and will diagnose most problems. Advanced imaging is required when there is something unusual about the problem or when the pain is associated with significant neurologic abnormalities. Failure to improve with conservative care is another indication for more extensive examination.

Causes of Neck Pain

As with the low back pain, most neck pain problems are benign and self-limited. Most appear to be muscular and ligamentous in origin. Myofascial pain appears to be an even greater component of neck pain syndrome than of low back pain. The most common cause of neck pain appears to be spondylotic degenerative disk disease. This may occur with or without nerve root compression and with or without stenosis. Neck pain also occurs as a complication of bone tumors or rheumatologic diseases such as rheumatoid arthritis, and may complicate neurologic diseases such as amyotrophic lateral sclerosis. Cervical spondylosis appears to be the most common syndrome.

Management of Cervical Pain

Acute episodes of neck pain usually associated with spasm and loss of range of motion are very common after unusual physical exertion, prolonged travel, or sleeping in an unaccustomed position. These acute problems usually disappear without evaluation or treatment. Treatment consists of adequate analgesia, usually with anti-inflammatory drugs or with mild narcotics, application of heat or cold as the patient prefers, and short-term restriction of activities. Many patients find massage produces short-term relief. Most acute pain will improve within 1 week and dissipate within 1 month.

Complaints associated with significant radicular pain, neurologic complications, or unusually severe pain may require more evaluation. This is always a matter of judgment and no strict rules apply. However, because neurologic function in the upper extremities is so critical, patients with sensory loss or sensory complaints involving the hand, or with any dysfunction of motor power in the upper extremities, or with severe radicular pain, should be evaluated immediately for the cause with x-rays and MRI.

The Persistent Cervical Syndrome

When pain does not remit spontaneously, active therapy may be required. However, there are even less data about physical therapy measures and manipulation for cervical disease than exist for the low back. But many clinicians believe that therapy measures are more effective for the neck than for a similar lumbar syndrome. The usual protocol consists of home traction, a range-of-motion exercise program, and the use of heat and massage for relief of muscle spasm.

Traction is generally applied over a door. I prefer light weights of 3 to 5 lb applied for fairly short periods (20 to 45 minutes). Using an over-the-door traction allows the patient to watch television, read, or be involved in other activities, rather than exclusively lying in bed. Most beds are not appropriately designed for the use of home traction, whereas the over-the-door system can be set up anywhere, even at work. Pain in the jaws or exacerbation of neck pain usually mean the weights are too heavy or the patient is staying in the traction too long.

The traction is supplemented by an exercise program that gradually puts the neck through full range of motion in all directions. As soon as the acute pain is gone, I begin an isometric exercise program in which the patient attempts to move his or her head in all directions against resistance. There are many illustrated descriptions of these exercises available commercially and I keep a supply of these books to give to patients.

Heat, massage, ultrasound, and transcutaneous electrical stimulation are all useful to relieve specific areas of muscle tightness and inflammation. A short course of anti-inflammatory medication is helpful. Some therapists employ trigger-point injections, which are indicated if specific severely painful trigger points can be identified.

Patients need to be reassured that these simple measures will take time to be effective so they do not become discouraged when relief is not immediate. In my experience, most patients can be maintained with these simple measures, and surgical intervention is not often required.

Severe Persistent Cervical Pain

When pain is severe and/or associated with neurologic complications, and is not relieved by time or conservative measures, surgical intervention may be required. When pain is radicular and unilateral, it is probably the result of nerve root compression, and simple decompression will be adequate to relieve the problem. When the pain involves only the neck it is much more difficult to manage. Surgery corrects only nerve root compression and instability. Unless one or the other is demonstrated, it is unlikely that surgery will be of value. Cervical spinal stenosis involving the canal compresses the spinal cord and produces myelopathy, not pain. Pain comes from movement and from pressure on the nerves.

When patients have not improved with conservative measures and surgery is contemplated, cervical x-rays and an MRI are adequate to make the diagnosis for most patients. The x-rays will disclose the bony abnormalities while the MRI will determine the status of the disks and spinal cord, nerves, and other soft tissues. A diagnosis is virtually always made with these techniques.

Operations on the Cervical Disk

The most straightforward operations are cervical diskectomy and cervical foraminotomy. These operations are analogous to simple lumbar diskectomy and require general anesthesia for most patients. A small midline incision is made over the spinous processes at the appropriate interspace and the paravertebral muscles are elevated from spine and laminae. A small keyhole is made to expose the nerve. If a true disk herniation is present, the disk can be removed. But if the problem is bony spurring, then the foraminotomy is adequate. Success rates of 95% and greater have been achieved by virtually all experienced surgeons when the operation is done for the appropriate indications. Normal function returns to patients promptly and they suffer no long-

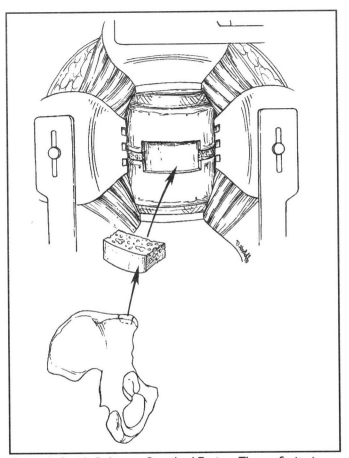

Figure 1: Smith-Robinson Standard Fusion. The graft site in the anterior superior iliac crest. The graft is formed to be placed in the disk space where the disk was removed.

term effects. Recurrence is rare. These straightforward operations are useful only for the specific unilateral radicular syndromes described and will not benefit the patient with a substantial degree of neck pain.

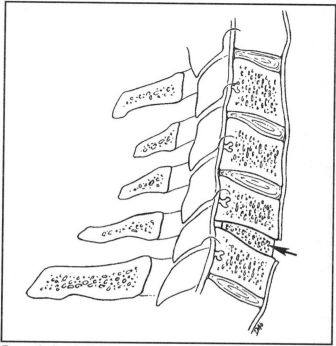

Figure 2: Smith-Robinson Standard Fusion. The graft is shown on lateral view replacing the disk between two vertebral bodies, as designated by the arrow.

When pain is bilateral, or when the arm pain is associated with considerable neck pain, the usual surgical approach is by the anterior route. The disk or disks to be removed are exposed by an anterior incision, and a route is taken just medial to the sternomastoid muscle. This allows the anterior surface of the disk or disks to be identified. They can be completely removed using this approach.

Many surgeons recommend only the diskectomy without the more traditional anterior fusion when radicular pain is the only problem. When neck pain is a large part of the syndrome, fusion is usually performed. The most popular fusion techniques are named for the surgeons who described them. The Smith-Robinson fusion uses the patient's own iliac crest or a similar block of bank bone to provide a plug, which replaces the disk that was removed (Figures 1 and 2). The Cloward technique requires removal of a dowel of bone from the cervical spine with a specially made drill and replacement with a similar dowel of bank or autologous bone harvested with a similar drill. The goal of both operations is eventual bony union across the interspace or the fusion of interspaces. A failure rate of fusion decreases the success of this operation, as contrasted with the posterior operations, but the indications are essentially different.

Increasingly, anterior fusions of more than one level are reinforced by an anterior plate-and-screw system that strengthens the neck and provides immediate stability. This has substantially decreased the failure rate of fusion.

Severe degrees of bony deformity do occur in the cervical spine. They are more dangerous than similar deformities in the low back because they are more severe and because they affect the spinal cord. Severe kyphosis produces spinal compression and myelopathy, as will any significant degree of instability. While these deformities require major reconstructive surgeries, they usually present with neurologic problems, not pain.

The Problem Patient Without Localizing Signs

Unfortunately, many patients with cervical spondylotic disease have diffuse complaints of neck pain without a radicular component to help localize the problem. Such patients often have multiple levels of degeneration, but occasionally no significant abnormalities are apparent. When these patients have persistent complaints, their evaluation for a possible remediable cause becomes important. This is one of the most controversial areas of spinal surgery and pain medicine.

Suboccipital and Upper Cervical Pain With Headache

A large group of patients is typified by complaints of suboccipital pain with headache usually radiating up the back of the head in the midline or on the lateral side involving the ear, thus implicating the upper cervical segments. Frequently, no abnormalities are seen on either examination or imaging. The first thing to do with such patients is to be certain that conservative or medical management will not relieve the symptoms. Because the pain of so many patients is not relieved by conservative means, a few medical centers around the world have begun to investigate the possibility that surgery may benefit some of these patients. This is based on the concept of the dysfunctional cervical spinal segment. Such patients are studied by a combination of diagnostic blocks of the upper cervical disks, the upper cervical facets, and the cervical roots. When a pain-producing segment can be identified, cervical fusion is recommended. Some surgeons have added rhizotomy or removal of the dorsal root ganglion at C2. While isolated reports have indicated the success of these procedures, not enough data are available to recommend this approach as a standard of care for these patients.

Another even larger group of patients presents with general complaints of neck and shoulder pain without radicular radiation. Such patients typically have multiple levels of degenerative disk disease involving the mid and lower cervical spine. Again, the principle of evaluation is the same. But here, long usage has established diagnostic diskography and anterior cervical fusion as standard treatment in the minds of many. Painful disks are identified by provocative diskography, and surgery based on pain production is typical for those who use these techniques. Other surgeons believe this policy is fallacious and do not use diskography or recommend surgery for these patients. The argument is yet to be settled by definitive data from either side.

Use of Nerve Blocks and Provocative Diskography in the Cervical Spine

The principle of nerve block is that if blockade of a structure relieves pain, then it is probable that the structure is involved in the generation of the pain. Specific nerve roots in the cervical spine are blocked to verify that radiating pain comes from that segment. Blockade of the zygapophyseal joints is much more complicated than nerve block in the cervical spine, but it can be done, and has been well-implemented by Bogduk. If blockade of a single segment relieves pain, it suggests that segment is the pain generator.

Provocative diskography is even more controversial than blockade. The diskogram was originally devised to determine the internal structure of the disk; then decisions for surgery were based on the demonstration of anatomical abnormalities. MRI has supplanted diskography for this purpose. It is now well recognized that pain syndromes do not necessarily correspond to degenerative disk disease. Now the practice of diskography is provocative so that the test is physiologic rather than simply anatomic. The disk is injected with saline and the pattern of pain recorded. If it conforms to the patent's usual pain, this is a positive test. The pain should then be relieved by the injection of a small amount of local anesthetic. When the patient's typical pain is provoked and relieved by injection of one or more segments, it is thought the painful segment or segments have been identified. Anterior cervical fusion is generally recommended. I believe that the data are not yet adequate to either accept or reject this concept.

Summary

The most important facts to recognize with neck pain are that most acute problems are self-limited and will disappear without therapy, and that medical management is all that is required for most persisting problems. Mild analgesics, exercise, and limitation of activities will usually make life tolerable for these patients. Surgery should be reserved for those in severe distress or with neurologic deficits, real or impending. Most patients will achieve excellent relief of radicular pain, but neck pain responds less well to surgical therapy. Surgery for isolated neck pain is still controversial.

References

1. Simeone FA, Rothman RH: Cervical disk disease. In: Rothman RH, Simeone FA, eds. *The Spine*. 2nd ed. Philadelphia, WB Saunders, 1982, pp 440-499.

Chapter 13

Pain in the Thoracic Spine

Thoracic spine pain is much less common than either low back pain or neck pain.[1] The supporting effect of the ribs undoubtedly contributes to the fact that degenerative pain is not as common here. Several specific syndromes are particularly troubling. The evaluation and management principles are the same as for low back pain. Unfortunately, the diseases of the thoracic spine tend to be much more serious and, therefore, generally require immediate attention when they do occur.

There is always a concern about confusing thoracic spine pain with visceral pain. A visceral syndrome rarely presents with thoracic spine pain and the patient's general complaints are more likely to lead to the diagnosis of visceral disease than to confusion with pain of spinal origin.[1]

Compression Fracture

A typical thoracic spine pain syndrome occurs in patients with osteoporosis when a vertebra partially collapses. Pain is local, although there may be some radiation around the chest from root compression if the collapse is severe. Then the pain follows the ribs. Unless neurologic deficit has occurred, clinical treatment options are few, such as recommending limitation of activities and prescribing analgesics. The pain continues for many months and may be permanent, although this is rare. Patients need to be reassured that the pain probably will disappear, but they must be resigned to the fact that months of discomfort may follow compression fracture. If neurologic deficit occurs, then surgical correction will be necessary. Otherwise, surgical repair has little function in this disease.

Thoracic Disk Herniation

Pain from thoracic disk herniation can be very severe. It is usually unilateral (although it may be bilateral), follows the root around the rib, and has a burning character. The great risk it poses is myelopathy. Patients should be carefully examined for hyperreflexia in the lower extremities, weakness, and Babinski signs. A sensory loss to the level of the herniation may also occur. Most patients with soft disk herniation will improve slowly. However, the risk of developing a deficit is much greater here because of the small canal and the proximity of the spinal cord. Patients can suddenly worsen. If the disk herniation is sizable and there is any sign of spinal cord compression, then immediate surgery is required. Most of these patients require a major procedure that includes removal of part of one rib by a transpleural or retropleural approach, excision of the disk, and fusion. While formidable, this operation is required when spinal cord compression occurs. When pain is the only issue, then it may be reasonable to wait for spontaneous remission. Severe pain that persists for 3 to 6 months will not disappear spontaneously.

Nonspecific Thoracic Spine Pain

Another large group of patients complain of axial pain more or less around the midline over specific segments of the thoracic spine. They do not have specific imaging finding, although osteoarthritic changes, disk calcification, and minor degrees of compression of vertebral bodies may be seen. These nonspecific complaints are also common in rheumatoid arthritis, ankylosing spondylitis, and similar diseases. The treatment is symptomatic.

A common related syndrome occurs in patients with minor degrees of scoliosis. Local pain is typical. These patients are usually treated with mild analgesics, anti-inflammatory drugs, and an exercise program to strengthen axial musculature. Fortunately, their complaints tend to be mild. Surgical fusion is not indicated for most of these patients.

References

1. North RB, Campbell JN, James CS, et al: Failed back surgery syndrome: 5-year follow-up in 102 patients undergoing repeated operation. *Neurosurgery* 1991;28(5):685-690.

WWWW *Chapter 14*

The Chronic Pain Syndrome and the Pain Treatment Center

Of all the pain problems, the chronic pain syndrome is the most difficult to manage. Patients are typically fixated on and completely disabled by the pain. Often involved in litigation, they commonly have a history of premorbid psychological dysfunction, often misuse narcotic and psychoactive medications, and use an inordinate amount of medical care.[1]

Features of the Chronic Pain Syndrome

Since spinal pain is second only to headache among all pain complaints, it is not surprising that spinal pain is the most common complaint for patients who fall into the chronic pain syndrome category.[2] However, virtually all diseases that cause pain can create the chronic pain condition. The syndrome is defined by more than chronic pain. First, these patients are incapacitated beyond any physical impairment. They are disabled by the complaint of pain alone. They fixate upon the pain to the exclusion of everything else in their life. Typically, these patients have a virtual pain neurosis.

Another characteristic is extensive use of the medical system. These patients have seen many physicians and undergone many interventions. Repeated diagnostic studies are common. Failed operations are the rule because often the indications for surgery were lacking and the operation was carried out for the complaint of chronic pain.

Drug misuse is common. These patients often take excessive amounts of narcotics and other psychoactive drugs, although true addiction with drug-seeking behavior is relatively rare. Patients often receive drugs from more than one physician and use them in amounts that are potentially harmful. Depression and anxiety are common, which most experts believe are reactive. However, both may be disabling and complicate management. Typically, such patients have the vegetative symptoms of depression, with difficulty sleeping and a predominately sedentary existence.

Pain behavior is also an important part of the syndrome patient. These patients moan and groan loudly with the slightest exertion. They often think that their pain has been worsened substantially by a simple physical examination, particularly if administered by an adverse physician in a litigation conflict. Patients often exert little or no effort on motor testing, but walk or stand without difficulty. An exaggerated limp and an inability to move from a chair or an examining table are common. They often nearly fall, but catch themselves before actually doing so. Complaints of sensory loss, distribution of pain, and patterns of motor loss are not anatomically and physiologically justified. The words they use to describe pain often suggest torture and are often emotion-laden, denoting suffering more than pain.

Patients often describe other physicians in pejorative terms and profess to believe that you are the best they have seen. They often say that you are their only hope.

Our extensive experience with these patients suggests that a relatively small number have overt psychiatric disease. Schizophrenia, endogenous depression, manic depressive disorder, and somatoform disorder are the most common. An equivalent number seem to have developed the chronic pain syndrome without an antecedent history of psychiatric disturbance. Most such patients exhibit personality vulnerabilities that existed before the pain-producing event. Careful historical evaluation suggests personality disorder or personality dysfunction. Those with true personality disorders are fewer than those who simply demonstrate vulnerabilities that have become important because of the stresses of the painful disease.

This constellation of problems means that patients can not only be treated for pain. All aspects of the syndrome require attention, and that is why the multidisciplinary pain treatment program evolved.

Evaluation of the Patient Exhibiting the Chronic Pain Syndrome

While the medical model of diagnosis and treatment does not suffice for most of these patients, it is important to begin with thorough diagnosis. Many of these patients have not had an adequate diagnosis and, therefore, have not had appropriate medical or surgical therapy. Begin with a complete and realistic diagnosis to identify any remediable cause of pain. Trivial abnormalities that could not explain the patient's incapacitation should not be given undue importance. These patients often have complaints in virtually every organic system. The careful physician must listen and choose those that have a reasonable chance of explaining the patient's pain or could be serious enough to warrant treatment. Every somatic complaint need not be evaluated thoroughly, nor does every new complaint require a new evaluation. This is a difficult judgment and such patients require a skilled physician. Unfortunately, the current disability litigation system often means they are evaluated by advocates for plaintiff and defendant positions. The plaintiff's physicians tend to find things no one else can find and emphasize trivial abnormalities that lead to unnecessary procedures and a countertherapeutic emphasis on maintaining symptoms. Defense physicians discount all complaints no matter how valid and emphasize psychosomatic aspects. They even deny valid diagnoses and attempt to withhold potentially curative treatments. The conscientious physician must avoid both traps. Medical evaluation and therapy should proceed as with any other patient, understanding that many of the chronic pain problems that seem so unusual are not unusual to the pain expert. If nothing obvious is forthcoming on routine examination, then referral to a pain expert is the next step.

The psychological/psychiatric assessment should be equally thorough. There is much misunderstanding about the role of psychiatric factors in pain problems. The psychiatrist is often asked, "Is the pain real?" Of course, no one can answer this but the pa-

Table 1: Signs of Addiction

Physicians should suspect addiction when the patient:

- exhibits drug-seeking behavior
- demands escalation of dose
- tries to get drugs from several physicians
- claims that only certain drugs "work"
- finds excuses for more drugs
- has serious side effects with abstinence

tient, who may, in fact, be malingering. The psychiatric evaluation seeks evidence of a diagnosable psychiatric condition. A thorough general physician can carry out a similar psychosocial examination that can be helpful in the overall assessment of patients. Judicious questions about work and recreation, marital status, education, work histories, status of litigation, and relations with others, will tell a great deal about the patient's personality vulnerabilities that must be considered when assessing the complaint of pain. Observation of pain behavior is another important issue. The presence of pain behavior does not imply psychiatric disease unless there is obvious exaggeration of behavioral disabilities. The importance of pain behavior has been assumed, but never proven. It may be that these naive patients are simply trying to impress upon skeptical physicians the importance of their complaint. Whatever the implications, it is apparent that pain behavior can be detrimental for these patients, so aberrations in behavior must be addressed.

The treatment for diagnosed psychiatric abnormalities should be typical for the disease. The presence of pain does not change appropriate therapy.

The next step is a careful drug history. The deleterious effects of narcotics and many psychoactive drugs are well known. Look for signs of addiction (Table 1), usually characterized by active drug-seeking behavior and steady escalation of dose. Patients get drugs from many different physicians and use a variety of stereotyped excuses to continue getting them.

Misuse is more common than addiction. Patients continue to escalate the dose until the amount of drug taken far exceeds that usually prescribed, and side effects become important. Patients are confused, exhibit mood disturbances, and lack judgment. Real withdrawal effects are common throughout the day as the frequent p.r.n. use of medication provides highs and lows. This combination of depression, anxiety, drug effect, and lack of activity can make such patients extremely dysfunctional.

The Multidisciplinary Pain Center

No single therapy is likely to benefit the patient exhibiting features of the chronic pain syndrome. Treating the pain is not enough, even when the treatment is straightforward. All aspects of the dysfunction, including those that are psychosocial, must be addressed. Recognizing these treatment needs led to the concept of the multidisciplinary pain treatment program. Consequently, the nonspecific nature of the pain complaint and the lack of effective treatment for many patients have led to the proliferation of self-styled pain treatment centers that lack expertise in diagnosis and treatment of pain.

To be an authentic pain treatment center, it must have these capabilities[1]: *(1) skilled diagnosis of the physical cause of the pain; (2) equally skilled psychological evaluation; (3) full range of therapies based on these diagnoses;* (4) *the capability to recognize drug misuse and to correct abuse of medications;* (5) *since physical inactivity is an important part of the disability these patients suffer, the center should have the capacity to recognize their needs and restore these patients to physical function. Many of these patients have managed to create complex disability-litigation situations that virtually preclude return to function; and (6) the capabilities to assist patients in correcting these social and vocational situations.*

Goals of Therapy

Most patients and their physicians naively assume that the goal of therapy is simply relief of pain. Unfortunately, many patients have problems for which there are no effective treatments. The first goal of a comprehensive center is to make the best diagnosis possible about the cause of pain and prescribe treatments most likely to alleviate the pain. Recognition and treatment of depression and anxiety are extremely important. Many patients can be restored to function, even if pain cannot be relieved. The deleterious effects of drug misuse must be corrected. Some patients may be candidates for long-term use of narcotics or for unusual procedures, such as spinal stimulation. These symptomatic therapies are rarely completely effective, but may make the patient substantially more functional. Protection from useless procedures that may be harmful, assistance with psychosocial problems, and improvement in function can all be beneficial.

Specific Treatment Programs in the Pain Treatment Center

Medications that do not have withdrawal potential should be ordered immediately and controlled. Patients should not misuse indicated medications, such as excessive use of narcotics. This control mechanism is usually done through a withdrawal program in which the narcotic is reduced 10% each day or every other day until it is eliminated. A new interest has emerged in investigating long-acting oral narcotics for relief of chronic pain of benign origin (see Chapter 10). Nevertheless, nearly all agree that short-acting narcotics, with their peaks and valleys of effect, are unsatisfactory for pain control in most of these patients. When long-term narcotic therapy is chosen, the long-acting narcotics (MS Contin®, Oramorph SR™, Duragesic®) are appropriate. Completing withdrawal first allows long-acting drugs to be established. The use of these drugs in chronic pain of benign origin is still unproven and is for now best left in the hands of experts.

A number of psychoactive drugs, particularly diazepam (Valium®), clonazepam (Klonopin®), and similar drugs, have withdrawal potential. Patients are withdrawn from them by reducing the dose 10% a day or every other day. Antidepression therapy can be instituted during withdrawal and will usually ameliorate the unpleasant side effects of withdrawing from this category of drugs. There is no evidence that one antidepressant has particular advantage over another. It is more important to find a drug that is well tolerated by the patient and has no side effects.

Stress Relief Techniques

Many patients find biofeedback, relaxation therapy, meditation, and individual counseling valuable techniques for the relief of stress. There is little evidence that any of these relieve pain, but they do make the patient more tolerant of pain and disability.

Behavioral modification can be valuable in managing these patients. Because pain behavior can be deleterious, patients need to change their focus from their pain and be convinced to function again. Many of them are sedentary for most of the day and need to be physically mobilized. Therefore, one important aspect of a behavioral modification program is to change physical capacities. Patients suffer the effects of inactivity and disuse. Local physical measures to improve range of motion and decrease myofascial pain are helpful. Physical reconditioning is important. While beyond the purview of the typical pain treatment program, vocational rehabilitation is helpful for many patients, especially those who have been unemployed for extended periods.

Behavioral therapy must go further than physical techniques, however. Many patients are convinced of the severity of their illness and their incapacitation. They must be re-educated to do the simplest things for themselves. Families need to be re-educated as well. Too often, oversolicitous family members are heavily invested in the disability syndrome. They often compound the problem by doing everything for the patient. All of those involved in the disability process need to understand what the patient can and cannot do, what will be harmful, and what will not. Behavioral techniques include community living and self-help while in the hospital, as well as formal education and rehabilitation programs. Removing fixation from drug therapy is an important part of behavioral change.

Alternative Therapies

Much is written and spoken enthusiastically in the support of alternative therapies for chronic pain. Acupuncture and manipulation therapy are commonly sought by patients, and the list of other therapy methods is long. In my view, there is no such thing as alternative medicine. There are therapy modes whereby efficacy has been established by appropriate studies in which a specified outcome is proven superior to the natural history of the disease. Some clinical questions can be examined by clinical trials. Data from these clinical trials constitute the best evidence of efficacy. Until the so-called alternative modes of therapy have been subjected to these kinds of reviews, they cannot be accepted, no matter how vocal their proponents may be. Remember the placebo-nocebo effect. We expect 10% of patients to be improved by any therapy for completely nonspecific reasons and, by the same token, 8% to 10% to believe they have been worsened. These figures have been verified as responses to sham therapies. Therefore, a small number of patients will think they have been dramatically improved by any treatment, no matter how nonspecific, and this must always be remembered in assessing anecdotal evidence of efficacy of therapy.

Many self-styled pain treatment centers have only one modality of treatment, such as therapeutic nerve block. The symptom of pain alone is treated without regard for underlying diagnosis. Claims of success are often exaggerated. Bona fide pain centers will have the capacity to deal with all legitimate therapies, although this does not imply that every patient needs every therapy available. Well-organized pain centers avoid reliance on a single mode of treatment, do not emphasize alternative modes of therapy, do not lack diagnostic capability, and avoid unrealistically optimistic claims for outcome.

For appropriate therapy, there must be a diagnosis, although seemingly bizarre, that can be common to the pain expert. The comorbidities that accompany chronic pain must be identified and treated. Those patients whose disease is not amenable to treatment must be offered symptomatic relief that includes therapy in all the areas of abnormalities. Therapy programs that have less than these capabilities are unlikely to help most patients.[1]

Psychological Aspects of Pain and Pain Therapy

Pain is a subjective experience recognized only by the individual who suffers the pain, but is more than the activation of sensory mechanisms. Pain has cognitive, affective, and behavioral components. Since the experience is personal, the pain therapist must use inferential measurements by interpreting what the patient reports and by observing the patient's behavior. Thus, the patient's experience of pain is modified by the therapist's experiences and prejudices. Pain behavior is the visible consequences of the pain as observed by others, and pain disability assesses the individual's ability to maintain active involvement in all of life's activities.[3,4]

A strong relation exists between pain and depression, but it is uncertain whether there is any true causative relationship.[5-7] My own data suggest that the chronic pain syndrome is more likely to develop in patients with psychiatric disease or personality vulnerability,[8] but not all clinicians agree. The depression found in patients suffering from chronic pain is usually reactive and responds well to medical therapies, in contrast to the more difficult endogenous depression in psychiatric patients. Pain behavior also correlates with depression, and both may be more an expression of depression than of any relationship to the severity of pain.[9]

Patients exhibiting chronic pain syndrome tend to give up responsibility for themselves, become dependent on the health-care delivery system,[10] and become passive. Many virtually attempt to turn over their lives to health-care professionals.

Patients suffering from chronic pain syndrome exhibit a state of anxiety. There is no evidence that trait characteristics are more common in patients who develop chronic pain syndrome, but it appears that the psychological profiles can be exacerbated by chronic pain. Patients tend to become more neurotic, hypochondriacal, and depressed, as measured by standard personality tests.

Generally, some patients are more vulnerable to stress, although clinicians disagree about whether these patients suffer from true personality disorder or have personality dysfunctions that are more easily disrupted by stress.

Patients with psychiatric disease exhibit increased complaints of pain, particularly patients with chronic anxiety syndromes, depression, or hysteria. A somatoform disorder is also commonly associated with complaints of pain in many organ systems.

The true hypochondriac, the conversion hysteric, and the somatization disorder patient all fall in this category. All perceive normal bodily functions as abnormal and apparently misinterpret many sensations as pain. Rarely, one encounters a true factitious disorder in which the patient deliberately creates the abnormalities.[6]

Schizophrenics will also occasionally complain of pain as a part of their disordered thinking.

In all these psychiatric diseases, appropriate treatment of the underlying disease, with relief of symptoms, will usually solve the pain complaint.

Psychological Therapies For Pain

The three psychiatric approaches to pain are: affective, cognitive, and behavioral.

Affective processes are the emotional reactions that occur with disease, tissue injury, and pain. The most common are anxiety, depression, and anger. Fear may also occur. Anger and fear particularly increase the distress associated with pain.

The cognitive processes include the amount of attention given to the pain and distraction. Involved are the patient's coping strategies, beliefs about the pain and its effects, previous painful experiences, and beliefs about the meaning of illness for the individual. Cognitive therapy focuses on the coping strategies that many patients have developed. They include distraction, attention diversion, imagery, and fantasy. Patients often feel helpless, even when helplessness is not a symptom of depression. Allowing them to gain control is an important issue.[11]

Behavioral abnormalities are basically pain behavior. Many patients create behavior patterns that aggravate the pain problem. They may cease to function in society, quit work, become sedentary, take excessive drugs, and reject their role as spouse, parent, or community member. Behavioral treatments include shaping and modeling positive behavior, reinforcing wanted behavior, and punishing negative behavior. Patients can be taught to do common things for themselves again. Physical conditioning is important. The goal is to substitute well behavior for pain, and functional behavior for disability.[12]

Family members and friends often must be included. The socialization of the patient often becomes distorted by the pain complaint, so it is important to reverse the sick role and bring family and friends into a supportive role that emphasizes well behavior.

Psychiatric and Psychological Treatments

The treatment of depression is usually medical. Patients respond well to oral antidepressants.[13] Amitriptyline (Elavil®) 25 to 100 mg given at bed time is an excellent drug and has a known beneficial effect on neuropathic pain in addition to its effect on depression. Other antidepressants have been less well studied for their pain effect, but are satisfactory for the treatment of depression. The individual practitioner should become familiar with some of these drugs.

Treatment of anxiety with antianxiety agents is also effective. Diazepam (Valium®) has the longest history. Because of its abuse potential, the use of this drug must be carefully monitored. Other drugs are satisfactory, and the physician should become knowledgeable about them while maintaining strict control of patient intake.

In addition to these medications, the general forms of psychotherapy can be useful,[14] including individual and group therapy, family therapy with appropriate support, and cognitive and behavioral techniques.

Supportive psychotherapy generally consists of ongoing reassurance, limited re-examinations to reinforce the reassurance, and redirection of interest for patients with chronic pain syndrome, somatoform disorders, or hypochondriasis.[15-18] An understanding physician or other health professional can usually keep these patients functional with limited re-evaluations that meet their needs but do not expose them to harm or to excessive cost.

It is usually valuable to interview a spouse or other relatives to be assured of the patient's veracity. Frequently, patient, spouse, or other close relatives can benefit significantly by frank discussions of the effect of chronic pain on personality, depression, and anxiety. Patients often simply need to be reassured that they will not harm themselves by increasing their activities. Restoring physical activity is an important part of this overall treatment plan.

Group therapies are the most effective. Long-term support groups appear to have considerable value in chronic pain.[14]

Generalist's Role in Psychiatric Care for Chronic Pain

Many of these features can be addressed by general and family physicians. If the symptoms are not severe, then the basic principles of therapy can be applied by any clinician. If the patient is seriously disabled, then psychiatric consultation and treatment are worthwhile. As soon as the patient is restored to reasonable function, maintenance therapy can generally be provided by a family physician, nurse, or support group, depending on the patient's needs.[19]

Behavioral Treatments

Many kinds of behavioral treatments are useful for patients with chronic pain. All of these attempt to teach the patient to take control and either lessen the perception of pain or reduce the negative influence of the pain on function.[20-23]

Many different forms of behavior treatments are available, such as relaxation strategies, whereby patients can be taught to relax tight muscles, reduce the apparent severity of the pain by autogenic training, and use biofeedback techniques. Biofeedback is a convenient way for patients to learn to control pain and other vegetative functions, and is an excellent technique for stress control. Some patients do well with hypnosis.

Cognitive strategies generally teach direct control of the pain and rational release of emotions.

Operant therapy basically rewards good behavior and punishes fixation on the pain. The patient is rewarded when the pain is controlled and when his or her behavior is functional.

These therapies all try to make the patient better able to cope with a pain state that cannot be treated otherwise. The goals are to minimize pain, increase adherence to the proposed therapeutic regimen, and increase function despite pain.

A fundamental part of all these treatments is trust between patient and therapist. The patient must be motivated to function better and the therapist must be committed to spending the time required to benefit the patient.

Most of these techniques require an expert for initial application. The multidisciplinary pain treatment center provides this constellation of psychologically based therapies and the experts who can administer them.

References

1. Long DM: A comprehensive model for the study of therapy of pain: Johns Hopkins Pain Research and Treatment Program. In: Ng LKY, ed. *New Approaches to Treatment of Chronic Pain: A Review of Multidisciplinary Pain Clinics and Pain Centers*. May, 1981, pp 66-75.

2. Long DM: Acute and chronic pain. In: Davis JH, Drucker WR, Foster RS, et al, eds. *Clinical Surgery*. Vol 1. St Louis, CV Mosby Co, 1987, pp 509-534.

3. Craig KD: Emotional aspects of pain. In: Wall PD, Melzack R, eds. *Textbook of Pain*. 2nd ed. Edinburgh, Churchill Livingstone, 1989, pp 220-330.

4. Waddell G, et al: Nonorganic physical signs in low back pain. *Spine* 1980;5:117-125.

5. Atkinson JH, et al: Depressed mood in chronic low back pain: relationship with stressful life events. *Pain* 1988;35:47-55.

6. Chaturvedi SK: Prevalence of chronic pain in psychiatric patients. *Pain* 1987;29:231-237.

7. Dworkin DH, Califor E: Psychiatric diagnosis and chronic pain: DSM-III-R and beyond. *J Pain Symptom Manage* 1988;3(2):87-98.

8. Turk DC, Flor H: Etiological theories and treatments for chronic back pain. II. Psychological modes and interventions. *Pain* 1984;19:209-233.

9. Edwards LD: Psychiatric, psychological and some physiological influences on the response to pain treatment: a review. *Methods Find Exp Clin Pharmacol* 1982;4:511-520.

10. Sternback RA: Clinical aspects of pain. In: Sternbach RA, ed. *The Psychology of Pain*. 2nd ed. New York, Raven Press, 1986, pp 223-239.

11. Turk DC, Rudy TE: Assessment of cognitive factors in chronic pain: a worthwhile enterprise? *J Consult Clin Psychol* 1986;54:760-768.

12. Fordyce WE: *Behavioral Methods for Chronic Pain and Illness.* S Louis, CV Mosby, 1976.

13. Goodkin K, Gullion CM: Antidepressants for the relief of chronic pain: do they work? *Ann Behav Med* 1989;11:83-101.

14. Gamsa A, Braha RED, Catchlove RFH: The use of structured group therapy sessions in the treatment of chronic pain patients. *Pain* 1985;22:91-96.

15. Ford CV: The somatizing disorders. *Psychosomatics* 1986;27:327-337.

16. Ford CV, Folk DG: Conversion disorders: an overview. *Psychosomatics* 1985;26:371-381.

17. Lipowski ZJ: Somatization: the concept and its clinical application *Am J Psychiatry* 1988;145:1358-1368.

18. Weisenberg M: Psychological intervention for the control of pain *Behav Res Ther* 1987;25:301-312.

19. Chapman CR, Turner JA: Psychological control of acute pain in medical settings. *J Pain Symptom Manage* 1986;1:9-20.

20. Fordyce WE, Roberts AH, Sternbach RA: The behavioral management of chronic pain: a response to critics. *Pain* 1985;22:113-126.

21. Keefe FJ, Gil KM: Behavioral concepts in the analysis of chronic pain syndromes. *J Consult Clin Psychol* 1986;54:776-783.

22. Turk DC, Meichenbaum D, Genest M: *Pain and Behavioral Medicine: A Cognitive Behavioral Perspective.* New York, Guilford Press 1983.

23. Turner JA, Chapman CR: Psychological interventions for chronic pain: a critical review. II. Operant conditioning, hypnosis and cognitive behavior therapy. *Pain* 1982;12:23-46.

Chapter 15

Narcotic Use In Chronic Pain of Benign Origin

The use of narcotic analgesia for acute pain, particularly postoperative pain, is well accepted. The new guidelines for management of cancer pain clarify long-term use of narcotics for patients with malignant disease. However, there is a mixed message concerning narcotic use in patients with pain of benign origin, which is unlikely to be improved by therapy or with time. Therefore, this approach requires some explanation.[1]

Use of Short-Acting Oral Narcotics in Chronic Pain of Benign Origin

Parenteral narcotics are not indicated in these patients. There is no difference in the analgesia achieved from equipotential drug doses of parenteral or oral narcotics. A patient with pain of benign origin who requires parenteral narcotics needs more than analgesia and should be suspected of addiction.

Most major pain treatment programs have determined that short-acting narcotics should be eliminated for pain of benign origin. Why? The principal reasons are these drugs' ineffectiveness for this kind of pain and their side effects. Some patients profess a need for short-acting oral narcotics to remain functional or to alleviate pain. However, in our experience at The Johns Hopkins Pain Treatment Center, detailing more than 1,000 of these patients, none received satisfactory pain relief from short-acting oral narcotics and not a single patient maintained function.

Negative side effects of these drugs include impaired cognition, inanition, accentuation of depression, mood changes (particularly irritability), constipation, and change in caloric intake.

True addiction must be considered a contraindication but evidence shows this is a problem in only a minority of patients. Virtually all of these patients are habituated to narcotic use, but do not exhibit .

All of these factors accentuate problems that are already being experienced by these patients. In addition, these patients may experience minor withdrawals throughout the day, coincident with rising and falling blood levels.

Withdrawal from short-acting narcotics has been a standard part of pain therapy for many years. Nearly all multidisciplinary programs require elimination of narcotics as a part of treatment. The experience at the Johns Hopkins Pain Center illustrates the point. Data from the withdrawal schedules of nearly 500 patients indicate that 10% of patients experienced substantial improvement in the pain complaint after withdrawal. In the rest, the pain remained stable. No patients studied thought their pain was worse after withdrawal.

Another issue related to long-term use of narcotic drugs is that many of them are combinations that include nonnarcotic analgesics known to be liver and kidney toxins. Therefore, the long-term ingestion of large amounts of acetaminophen, aspirin, or other related compounds may be harmful.

For all of these reasons, there is little enthusiasm for treatment of patients with chronic pain of benign origin with short-acting narcotics. This does not mean that the occasional judicious use of these drugs is unacceptable. Patients must be carefully chosen and drugs used episodically and sparingly.

Long-Acting Narcotics in the Treatment of Chronic Pain of Benign Origin

The advent of long-acting narcotics as effective oral agents has improved the management of cancer pain considerably. Naturally, the positive experience of managing cancer pain with these oral narcotics has led to the investigation of their use for pain of benign origin. The abuse potential of these drugs is small. They do not produce euphoria. They are habituating, but this habituation is a small price to pay if excellent pain relief improves function for these patients. Before describing how they are used, it is important to emphasize that the long-term success of these drugs for pain control is unknown, as are the potential side effects. The effects on cognition, other brain functions, liver, bowel, and kidneys certainly must be monitored. The use of these drugs for chronic pain of benign origin must be considered investigational at present and patients need to understand that the long-term consequences are not fully known.

Practical Use of Long-Acting Narcotics

Three forms of these drugs are now easily available and in widespread use for many purposes, mainly cancer pain. Methadone (Dolophine®) is an excellent oral analgesic, well absorbed and well tolerated. It has a long history for amelioration of heroin addiction, so more is known about its long-term consequences. It has two other advantages, one psychological and one economic. The psychological advantage relates to those who dispense the drug. Doses of methadone given orally conform to parenteral doses with which physicians, pharmacists, and nurses are familiar. Therefore, caregivers consider the doses reasonable. When other oral narcotics such as morphine sulfate are used, the doses seem to be extremely high to those who do not remember the low absorption rates and thus are less likely to provide adequate analgesic doses, fearing larger doses as dangerous. The other advantage is cost. Methadone is inexpensive, while other compounds are expensive. The principal negative feature of methadone is also psychological. Because most people have a vague understanding that it is used in drug withdrawal programs and forget that it is a potent analgesic, patients and health practitioners view methadone as implying treatment of addiction.

I begin with a relatively low dose of 6 mg to 12 mg given by mouth 4 times a day. The usual period of adequate analgesia with methadone is 6 to 8 hours, but as the drug rises in blood levels the dosage can be reduced to 3 times per day and then to twice a day. Some patients will do well with a single daily dose. Gradually escalate the dose until adequate analgesia is achieved. The usual side effects are confusion, sedation, general inanition, or severe constipation, which make it unpleasant for affected patients to continue the drug. Once achieved, a stable dosage should be maintained. Escalation and drug-seeking behavior have been rare problems.

The second popular form of long-acting narcotic are the morphine preparations (MS Contin®, Oramorph SR™). These drugs were developed specifically for oral administration. The major advantage is the duration of action. Dosages twice a day, even once a day, are reasonable. Some patients will achieve adequate relief with doses that are even less frequent. I begin with twice-a-day dosage. The goal is to achieve analgesia with the smallest amount of drug possible. A psychological drawback of this drug is that doses seem large. Patients may take hundreds of milligrams per day to get adequate analgesia. Clinicians who forget the low absorption rate of oral morphine are prone to think that patients are taking excessive doses of drug when only a small amount is actually absorbed into the blood. The goal is analgesia without side effects, so the actual dosage is not as important. There appears to be little abuse potential.

Typically, patients start at doses equivalent to or slightly greater than the amount of short-acting narcotic they are taking. If short-acting narcotics had not been used, then I usually begin at a small dose, 15 to 30 mg of morphine sulfate twice a day, observe how the drug is tolerated, and then escalate according to the patient's need.

The third common drug form now in use is administered by the cutaneous patch. Fentanyl is a potent analgesic that can be employed through the transdermal patch technique (Duragesic®). While effective and handy for the patient, patches had the historical disadvantage of being expensive but competitive pricing now makes them a cost-effective alternative. They are also an excellent way to achieve analgesia while switching a patient to a less expensive oral drug. The patches generally provide several days of pain relief after application and free the patient from a schedule of oral narcotics.

Table 1: Equianalgesic Conversion of Oral Opioids to Morphine Tablets

Current oral product	PO doses and schedule	Approximate equianalgesic regimen of morphine sulfate tablets
Morphine (MSIR®, Roxanol™)	10 mg q 4 h	2 tablets 15 mg q 12 h
	30 mg q 4 h	3 tablets 30 mg q 12 h
	80 mg q 4 h	4 tablets 60 mg q 12 h
	100 mg q 4 h	3 tablets 100 mg q 12 h
Hydromorphone (Dilaudid®)	4 mg q 4 h	3 tablets 15 mg q 12 h
	8 mg q 4 h	3 tablets 30 mg q 12 h
	10 mg q 4 h	2 tablets 60 mg q 12 h
	25 mg q 4 h	3 tablets 100 mg q 12 h
Methadone (Dolophine®)	10 mg q 6 h	2 tablets 15 mg q 12 h
	20 mg q 6 h	2 tablets 30 mg q 12 h
	30 mg q 4 h	2 tablets 60 mg q 12 h
	70 mg q 4 h	3 tablets 100 mg q 12 h
Meperidine (Demerol®)	100 mg q 3 h	2 tablets 15 mg q 12 h
	200 mg q 3 h	2 tablets 30 mg q 12 h
	600 mg q 3 h	2 tablets 60 mg q 12 h
	1000 mg q 3 h	3 tablets 100 mg q 12 h
Levorphanol (Levo-Dromoran®)	2 mg q 6 h	2 tablets 15 mg q 12 h
	4 mg q 6 h	2 tablets 30 mg q 12 h
	6 mg q 4 h	2 tablets 60 mg q 12 h
	14 mg q 4 h	3 tablets 100 mg q 12 h
Oxycodone (Roxicodone™)	10 mg q 4 h	2 tablets 15 mg q 12 h
	20 mg q 4 h	2 tablets 30 mg q 12 h
	40 mg q 4 h	2 tablets 60 mg q 12 h
	100 mg q 4 h	3 tablets 100 mg q 12 h

After stabilization, reduce the number of tablets, changing to the appropriate tablet strength: 30-mg, 60-mg, or 100-mg tablets q 12 h.

(Adapted and printed with permission of the Purdue Frederick Co., Norwalk, CT.)

The side effects are the same as for any other narcotic. Elderly people seem to have a greater tendency to develop cognitive deficits when using the transdermal patches.

Another common use of the patch is in the progression of drug use when the patient is beginning long-acting oral narcotics. One common technique is to bring the patient into the hospital and begin patient-controlled analgesia with small doses of drug to determine how much the patient needs for adequate pain relief. This can be accomplished in 2 or 3 days. Then a transdermal patch is applied, based on the doses needed, and continued while the patient begins a small dose of oral narcotics, which then escalates as patch use is discontinued. This is a technique that requires some experience, but is an efficient way to bring a patient to an adequate level of analgesia quickly.

Conversion formulas for typical short-acting and oral narcotic analgesics to morphine tablets are found in Table 1.

References

1. Payne R, Foley KM, eds: *The Medical Clinics of North America: Cancer Pain*. Philadelphia, WB Saunders Co, 1987.

Chapter 16

Management of Pain in Arthritis

P ain is a common symptom of arthritic disease and may accompany osteoarthritic change in a single joint or may be a symptom of widespread joint disease. Some specific syndromes should be recognized by the pain they produce. The treatment is mostly symptomatic. The most important issues are recognizing the rheumatologic diseases, choosing appropriate pain relief therapy, and being certain that patients are protected from joint injury when adequate analgesia is achieved.[1,2]

Diagnosing the Inflammatory Arthritic Syndromes

Rheumatoid Arthritis. This disease occurs three times more often in females than in males. There is usually symmetrical joint involvement beginning with, and particularly affecting, wrists and fingers. Subcutaneous nodules are frequently found over bony prominences. X-rays demonstrate osteoporosis near joints, loss of cartilage, and articular erosions. Remember, the disease often affects the spine, and patients can develop myelopathy from craniocervical instability.

Ankylosing Spondylitis. This disease occurs in males by a 7-to-1 ratio. It begins in the sacroiliac joints and ascends the spine sequentially. The bamboo sign seen on plain x-rays is diagnostic. Remember, these patients may develop aortic insufficiency and iritis.

Juvenile Arthritis. This disease is similar to rheumatoid and ankylosing diseases but serology studies will be normal. There is a predilection for the cervical spine, where the onset is acutely inflammatory.

Psoriatic Arthritis. Patients with psoriasis often have widespread arthritic change similar to rheumatoid disease. The arthritic disease may occur before the skin lesions, which confirm the diagnosis. Serology will be negative.

Reiter's Syndrome. This disease is characterized by an asymmetric involvement of the joints, beginning in the lower extremities. Spondylotic changes in the spine are common. The disease is associated with urethritis, infectious diarrhea, conjunctivitis, iritis and, occasionally, with skin lesions.

Behcet's Syndrome. This is similar to Reiter's syndrome, but the eye involvement is more obvious, and the arthritis is usually asymmetrical.

Infectious Arthritis. The infection usually involves one joint, but multifocal infectious arthropathy is possible. Septicemia may lead to heart valve colonization.

Lyme Disease. Lyme disease is particularly common on the East coast. A spirochetal infection, it usually causes a characteristic skin rash that precedes the arthritis. However, arthritic pain is the most important common feature of the early stages of the disease. Heart involvement comes next, and then neurologic symptoms occur as a third stage.

Rheumatic Fever. Rheumatic fever used to be a serious threat, but has virtually disappeared in the United States. There is a preceding group A streptococcal infection. Serologies will be positive. It has a predilection for cardiac valvular disease. Chorea may also occur. Migratory polyarthritis is common.

Degenerative Osteoarthritis. The most common form of arthritis, it characteristically involves the hand, the first metacarpal phalangeal joint, and distal joints. Major joints, such as knees and hips, are most severely affected. It is not related to spinal spondylosis.

Metabolic Arthritis. The typical metabolic arthritic problem is gout. This occurs more in males by a 10-to-1 ratio. It usually affects single joints, with the attacks being self-limited, typically lasting 4 to 7 days. Tophi appear in the ear and around joints. The diagnosis is made by an elevated uric acid, and by the aspiration of uric acid crystals from joints.

Similar diseases, such as pseudogout and ochronosis, are rare.

Connective Tissue Syndromes

The connective tissue diseases—lupus, scleroderma, and dermatomyositis—all present with joint pain. Lupus characteristically has a significant arthropathy, which may appear early in the disease. Scleroderma is less likely to have arthropathy, and more likely to present with Raynaud's syndrome. Nevertheless, an arthropathy can occur. Dermatomyositis presents with muscle weakness, atrophy, and polymyositic pain.

The evaluation and treatment of each of these diverse syndromes are beyond the scope of this book. Because the patient complaining of pain may harbor one of these unusual diseases, an evaluation of these arthritides should be included in every pain workup. The physician should think about them and examine clinical evidence for them.

The issue in all of these syndromes is how the pain should be treated. In general, pain treatment should start with treatment of the underlying disease. Once the disease is treated appropriately, then analgesics can be used if pain persists. The rules remain the same. Begin with nonsteroidal anti-inflammatory drugs (NSAIDs), which are particularly useful in most of these syndromes (see Table 1 in Chapter 4). When treatment of the underlying disease and the NSAIDs are ineffective, mild narcotics may be useful. It is rare that treatment of the primary disease and the use of NSAIDs are not satisfactory for pain control in these syndromes.[1,2]

References

1. Beary JF, Christian CL, Johanson NA: *Manual of Rheumatology and Outpatient Orthopedic Disorders*. 2nd ed. Boston, Little Brown and Co, 1987.

2. Kelley WN, et al: *Textbook of Rheumatology*. 3rd ed. Philadelphia, WB Saunders Co, 1989.

Index

irritability 180
Isoptin®, Knoll 100

J

Johns Hopkins Pain Treatment Center 136, 179

K

ketoprofen 34
    see Orudis®
ketorolac tromethamine 34
    see Toradol®
Klonopin®, Roche 28, 99-103, 170
kyphosis 58, 159

L

lacrimation 116
lactose 22
Lamictal®, Glaxo Wellcome 100
laminae 56, 80, 83, 156
laminectomy 24, 48, 50, 80-84, 89
Lanoxin®, Glaxo Wellcome 100
laser 84
lateral translation 86
leg extension 62
lemniscus 18
lemon 113
Levo-Dromoran®, Roche 34, 36, 40, 100, 183
levorphanol 34, 36, 40, 44, 183
    see Levo-Dromoran®

lidocaine 101
    see Decadron®;
    Xylocaine®
ligament hypertrophy 55
ligamentous inflammatory disease 53
ligamentum flavum 81
lima beans 113
limbic system 14, 15, 18
Limbitrol®, Roche 100, 102, 103
lime 113
limitation of activities 7, 8, 161, 162
Lissauer's tract 17
lithium carbonate 119
Lodine®, Wyeth-Ayerst 32, 100, 102
Lorcet®, Forest 38, 40, 100
Lortab®, UCB 38, 40, 100
lumbar disk 54, 57, 77, 81, 83, 84, 89
lumbar fascia 56
lumbar instability 59
lumbar spine 56, 62, 77, 85, 86, 89, 90
lumbosacral fusion 85
lumbosacral plexus 28, 95
lumbosacral spine 57, 62, 90
lumbosacral strain (or sprain) 54
lupus 187
Lyme disease 186

M

Magan®, Savage 34

nerve root compression 58-61, 66, 67, 69, 70, 73-75, 78, 90, 95, 154, 156, 162
nerve root irritation 57
nervus intermedius 48
neuralgia
  glossopharyngeal 106, 107
  postherpetic 97, 99, 103, 107, 125, 126
  trigeminal 51, 103, 106, 107, 148, 149, 150
neuroma 96, 103, 131, 143, 144
Neurontin®, Parke-Davis 100-103
neuropathic syndrome 28, 95
neuropathy 28, 58, 66, 95, 104, 125, 126, 130-132
neurotomy 144, 145
nifedipine 102
  see Adalat®; Procardia®
nitrates 112
nociceptive system 27
nociceptors 14, 16, 17
  A delta 14, 16, 17, 20
  C 14, 16, 17
  sleeping (or silent) 16, 17
nonsteroidal anti-inflammatory drugs (NSAIDs) 30, 32-35, 100, 106, 108, 119, 124, 127-129, 187
Norpace®, Searle 100
Norpramin®, Hoechst Marion Roussel 100, 102, 103

nucleotomy 84
nucleus pulposus 54, 56, 57
numbness 60, 73, 75
Nutrasweet® 113
nuts 112

O

ochronosis 187
odynophagia 126
olivary nucleus 18
Ondine's curse 50
onions 113
operant therapy 176
opiates 5, 19, 20, 24, 100, 102
opioids 19, 20, 22, 30, 35-41, 43, 45, 46, 119, 127-130
  agonists 20, 36, 40
  intramuscular 39
  oral 38, 129, 183
  parenteral 39
  receptors 19, 20
  short-acting 45
  transdermal 39
oral bioavailability 22
Oramorph SR™, Roxane 22, 34-36, 40, 100, 102, 107, 125, 134, 182
orange 113
oropharynx 109, 110
Orudis®, Wyeth-Ayerst 34
osteoarthritis 111, 186
osteoporosis 8, 162, 185
overdose 23

NOTES

NOTES